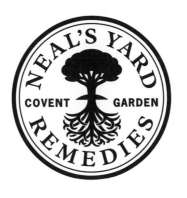

COMPLETE
MASSAGE

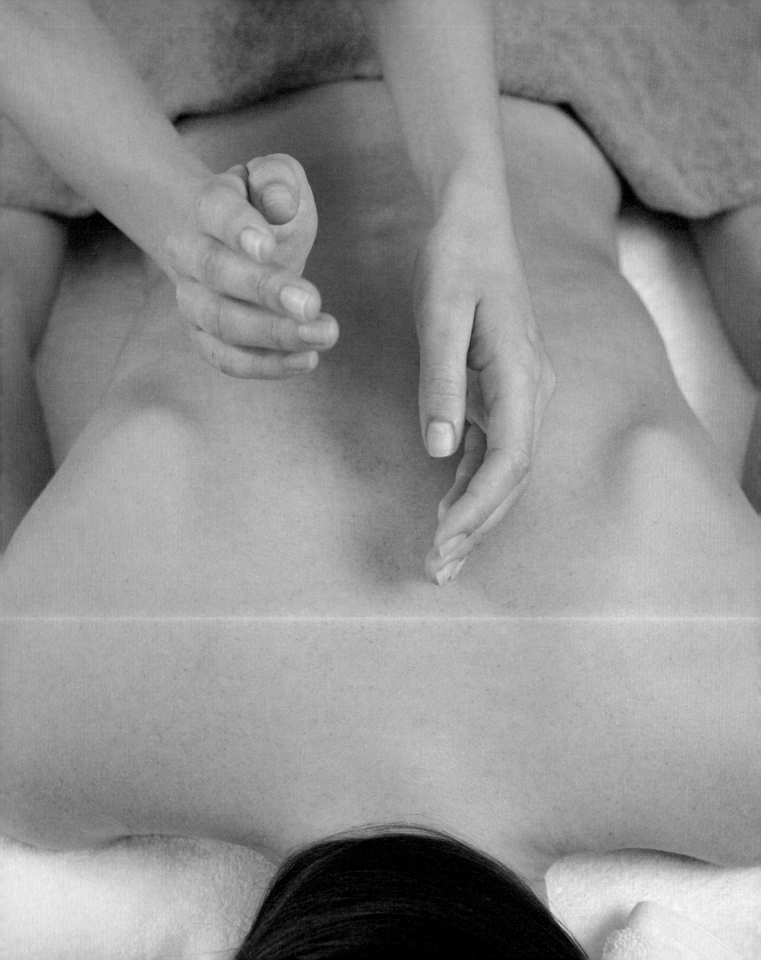

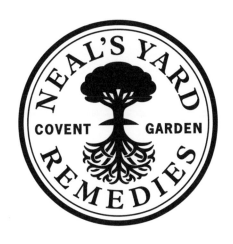

COMPLETE
MASSAGE

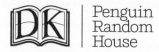

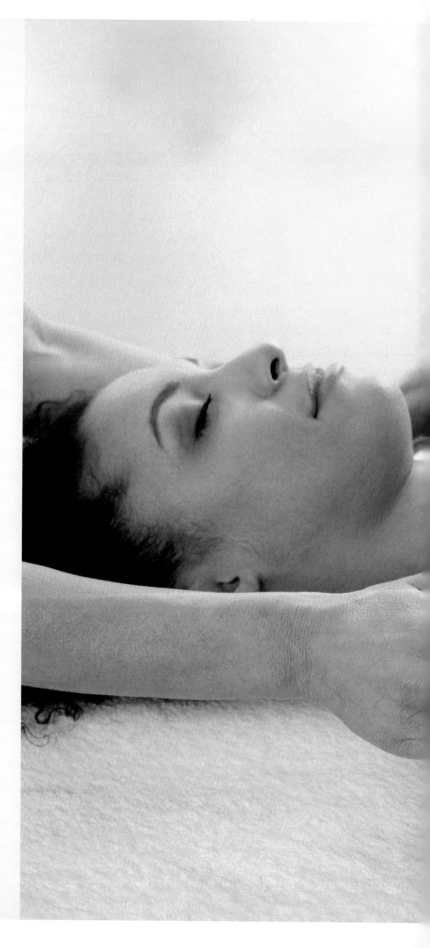

Senior Editor Claire Cross
Project Art Editor Louise Brigenshaw
Editorial Assistants Megan Lea, Kiron Gill
US Editor Kayla Dugger
Designers Vanessa Hamilton, Saskia Janssen, Sophie State
Illustrator Ryn Frank
Photographer Nigel Wright
Photography Production XAB Design
Producer, Pre-Production Heather Blagden
Producer Luca Bazzoli
Senior Jacket Creative Nicola Powling
Jacket Coordinator Lucy Philpott
Creative Technical Support Sonia Charbonnier
Managing Editor Dawn Henderson
Managing Art Editor Marianne Markham
Art Director Maxine Pedliham
Publishing Director Mary-Clare Jerram

First American Edition, 2019
Published in the United States by DK Publishing
1450 Broadway, Suite 801, New York, NY 10018

Copyright © 2019 Dorling Kindersley Limited
DK, a Division of Penguin Random House LLC
19 20 21 22 23 10 9 8 7 6 5 4 3 2 1
001–313753–Sep/2019

DISCLAIMER See page 252

A catalog record for this book is available from
the Library of Congress.

ISBN 978-1-4654-8394-2

Printed and bound in China

All images © Dorling Kindersley Limited.
For further information see: www.dkimages.com

A WORLD OF IDEAS:
SEE ALL THERE IS TO KNOW

www.dk.com

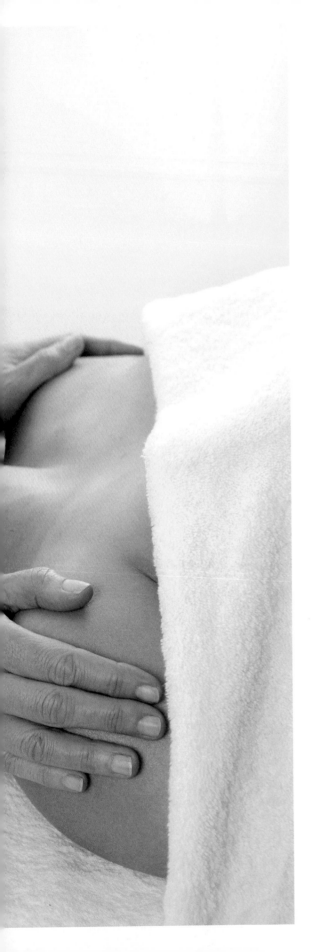

THE AUTHORS

Victoria Plum is the consultant editor for the book. She has been an aromatherapy and massage practitioner since 1996 and feels there is still so much to learn. Victoria specializes in the field of mental and emotional health, which developed and refined her hands-on work and led her to train as a craniosacral therapist. She is also a reiki practitioner. She taught for the Tisserand Institute from 1999. When the school closed in 2005, she was invited to teach courses for Neal's Yard Remedies. She believes that practice and teaching the practice feel like mutually inspiring and beneficial activities.

Nicola Leighton is a professional aromatherapist and massage therapist, having originally trained with Neal's Yard Remedies. She uses her knowledge of aromatherapy and advanced massage techniques, such as trigger point therapy, to treat the clients in her busy Cambridge clinic effectively. Nicola loves supporting people in all stages of life, finding the tools to help them thrive both physically and emotionally.

Fran Johnson is a passionate cosmetic scientist and aromatherapist and has been part of the Product Development team at Neal's Yard Remedies since 2006, formulating therapeutic products for healing and well-being. She has written for and teaches a number of Neal's Yard Remedies' courses, which cover aromatherapy, natural perfumery, and making cosmetic products.

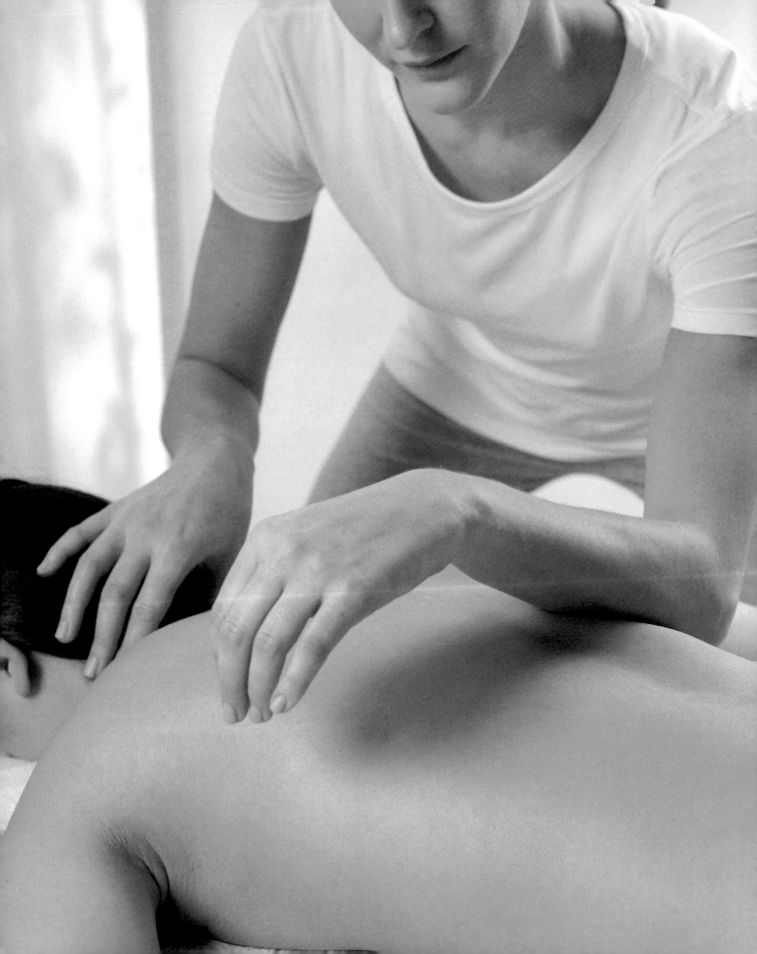

CONTENTS

FOREWORD

Hippocrates, the "father of medicine," said about massage and its importance as a skill for doctors that, "The physician must be experienced in many things, but assuredly in rubbing." Massage, he maintained, could loosen tightness, but also add tone where there was coldness and weakness in muscles. Depending on the speed and type of strokes used, massage could also calm and relax or invigorate and energize.

Medical texts dating back thousands of years from regions such as India, China, and Egypt provide instruction on massage and talk of its role in the maintenance of health and well-being.

The practice of massage should not be viewed as an ancient, charming superstition though. There is plenty of hard evidence showing the importance of touch, particularly in mammals. "Massage" performed by a mammalian tongue as it cleans its newborn kick-starts the healthy functioning of several body systems, while studies carried out on delicate premature babies show that the babies who were gently stroked in their incubators reached a normal newborn weight more rapidly than the babies who received just the essential medical care. We are kinesthetic creatures, innately aware of our bodies and how they are moving. The skin is our largest sense organ. Even our language shows that the quality of a touch can have a profound effect on us. When positively moved by another, we say that their words, gestures, or actions touch us, while a negative, scary, or suspicious presence may "make our flesh crawl."

The kindness of touch is something we instinctively offer each other—and ourselves. We rub our own tight muscles, our painful head when we have a headache, or our limbs to relieve the pain when we bang into objects. For others, we use touch to console, instinctively stroking the shoulder or arm of a friend, child, parent, or lover who is distressed. This kind of touch says "I see you, I hear you, and I care."

"The kindness of touch is something we instinctively offer each other, and ourselves, to soothe, ease pain, and console."

However, in a world where connections are increasingly virtual and we are used to being spoken to by automated voices, we are less and less comfortable with the messy, wonderful stuff of being human. Of course, not all touch is welcome, but the fear of inappropriate touch and the replacement of human transactions by ones between human and machine are closing down our capacity to touch and be touched in a way that connects us to our own humanity.

Massage is a mutual activity, not just something that one person—the giver—does to another—the receiver. If we massage someone's back with our hand or forearm, their back, in turn, massages our hand or forearm. Who is giving and receiving kindness here? Who is listening to and speaking through the quality of touch?

The art—and science—of rubbing is, of course, a technical skill that we may want to perfect and, indeed, need to if we want to be massage practitioners. With this book, we hope to inspire, educate, and empower. It offers a "toolkit" of techniques and treatment ideas for those just starting out, and may inspire experienced therapists to explore further training. Equally, and maybe even more importantly, we hope it will inspire the nonprofessional to oil up their hands to soothe a friend's aching shoulders, calm their baby's colic, relieve their own sore calves, or brighten their tired face with self-massage rather than rubbing in face cream!

It isn't just physicians who can benefit from the art of massage—it is all of us!

Victoria Plum

GETTING STARTED

Massage is so much more than a set of techniques. To appreciate the complexity of the practice and put your massage into context, a knowledge of key body structures and systems and consideration of how to prepare will give your practice depth and purpose. Here, a brief introduction to anatomy and physiology provides a handy starting reference, while an overview of aromatherapy shows the therapeutic possibilities for combining this holistic art with massage. Tips and checklists ensure you are equipped and physically and mentally ready. Most importantly, a guide to safe practice provides essential advice to protect both you and the receiver and ensure you practice with integrity.

THE BENEFITS OF MASSAGE

Touch is a basic and powerful human instinct that has the ability to reassure and comfort. Massage therapy uses touch not only to relax the whole body, but also to provide a range of therapeutic health benefits—primarily for the receiver, but also for the giver. Each treatment works holistically to bring relief and release to both the body and mind, promoting an overall sense of increased well-being.

HOW MASSAGE HELPS THE BODY

Massage therapy has a range of benefits for the body. On a physiological level, it helps improve the functioning of the body's systems (see pp.18–23), and it is also used to target specific conditions and relieve their symptoms.

One of the most notable benefits of massage is the stimulating effect that manipulating tissues has on the circulation of blood and lymph, which in turn helps oxygenate tissues all over the body, distribute nutrients to each cell, and support the efficient removal of waste. The increase in local circulation to the area that is being massaged also has a warming effect that relieves muscular tension and chronic pain. Overall, an improved circulation can have a profound impact on our health and well-being.

The relaxing effects of massage also support healthy blood pressure, and the release of tension in the body stimulates and strengthens the immune system, helping build resistance to illness and increase its ability to ward off infections.

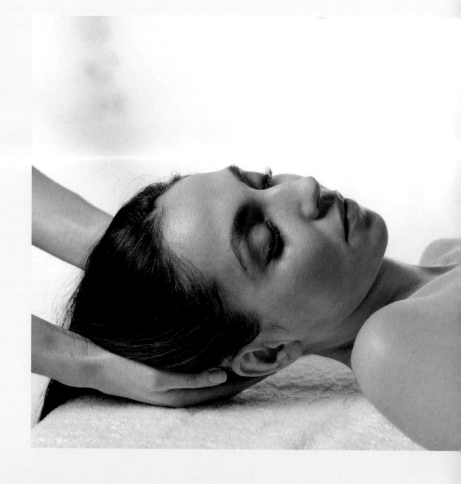

Another key benefit of massage is its ability to increase mobility and flexibility. By improving muscle tone and body awareness and stretching tissues, massage improves mobility; enhances athletic performance; and improves posture, which in turn ensures that internal organs have sufficient space to function optimally.

Massage can also be used to target specific complaints. For example, certain techniques can help reduce congestion in the lungs and improve lung capacity by relaxing tightness in the respiratory muscles. Also, working on the abdominal area can support digestion by improving the process of peristalsis— the wavelike contractions that pass waste through the large intestine. This in turn helps relieve the symptoms of gas, constipation, and also colic in babies.

STAYING WELL

Importantly, massage also acts as a preventative tool. By easing muscular tension and aiding relaxation, massage can help prevent physical pain and also release psychological tension and emotions that can manifest as physical symptoms.

DEEP RELAXATION
Massage is a truly holistic treatment, relaxing both the body and mind to help heal the body and improve well-being.▼

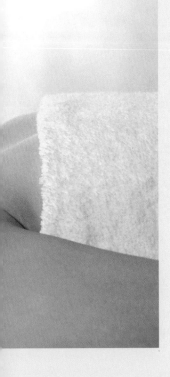

"The holistic benefits of massage can have a profound effect on health and well-being for both giver and receiver."

A HOLISTIC PRACTICE

Looking after our emotional health is increasingly important in today's hectic world. Prioritizing time out to recharge both mind and body and replenish our natural resources is key for balancing energy throughout the body and managing stress.

Not only does massage have a naturally uplifting effect—in part because touch boosts the body's levels of oxytocin, serotonin, and dopamine, the feel-good hormones—but it can also improve self-esteem; promote a sense of balance and harmony in body and mind; and provide effective relief from stress. All of these factors can ease the symptoms of anxiety and depression, in turn promoting good-quality, restful sleep and providing a sense of comfort that leads to enhanced well-being.

BENEFITS FOR THE PRACTITIONER

The powerful effects of massage bring benefits to both giver and receiver. As a practitioner, massage can develop into a deeply meditative practice as you learn how to enter into a state of focused relaxation, both to enhance your own practice and to model the deep relaxation that you are encouraging in the receiver. In this way, using the power of touch in massage promotes a feeling of inner calm and increased well-being that can carry over into everyday life.

Massage is also mentally stimulating as a practitioner as you enjoy the fulfillment that is gained through learning and refining skills. Physically, you need to learn how to improve posture, distribute weight correctly, and move around with fluidity to avoid damaging your own body, all of which will have an extremely positive and lasting impact on your overall health and well-being.

UNDERSTANDING THE BODY

A basic knowledge of anatomy and physiology puts massage in context. Understanding the musculoskeletal system—the location of muscles and how these attach to bones and joints—is key. Also, an awareness of how other body systems work, the structure of skin, and the positioning of major organs will help inform your practice.

MUSCULOSKELETAL SYSTEM

The body has two types of muscle. Involuntary muscle, such as heart muscle, is not under our immediate conscious control. Voluntary, or skeletal, muscles—for example, in the legs—are the ones we move by will. Skeletal muscle is composed of muscle and nerve fibers, bound together by connective tissue, and is attached to bones by fibrous tendons. Together with the skeleton, muscles give shape to the body and facilitate movement.

Muscles work in pairs, responding to signals from the brain. Fibers slide over each other during a contraction as a muscle shortens; as the muscle contracts, providing movement, the opposing muscle relaxes, providing stability and balance.

THE EFFECT OF MASSAGE

Muscles need oxygen and glucose to work efficiently and expel waste such as lactic acid, produced during vigorous or prolonged exercise. If muscles aren't relaxed sufficiently, waste builds up, slowing the circulation and

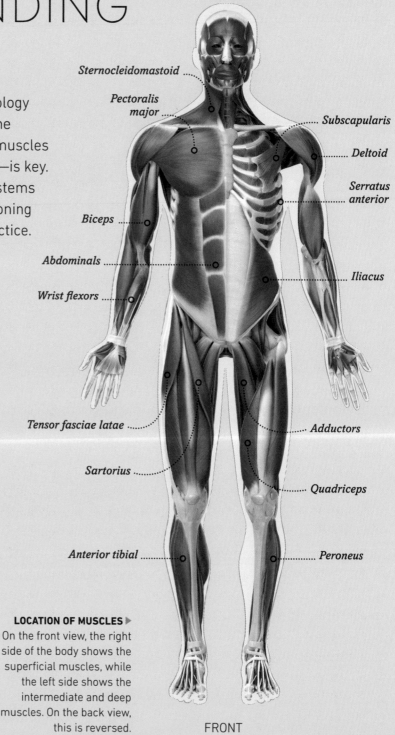

Sternocleidomastoid

Pectoralis major

Subscapularis

Deltoid

Serratus anterior

Biceps

Abdominals

Iliacus

Wrist flexors

Tensor fasciae latae

Adductors

Sartorius

Quadriceps

Anterior tibial

Peroneus

LOCATION OF MUSCLES ▶
On the front view, the right side of the body shows the superficial muscles, while the left side shows the intermediate and deep muscles. On the back view, this is reversed.

FRONT

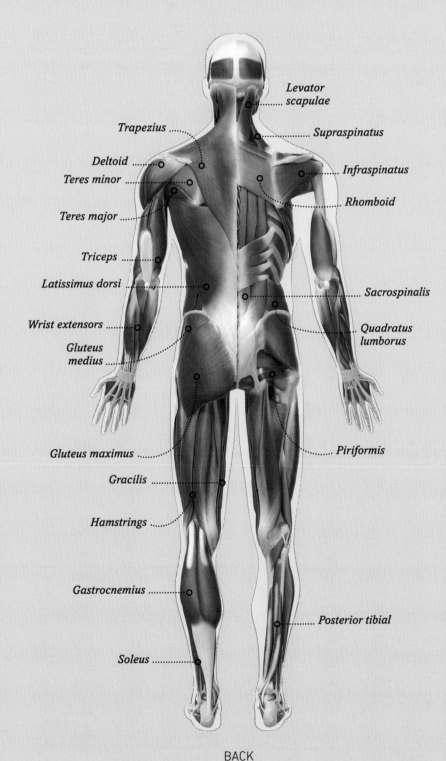

Levator
scapulae

Trapezius

Supraspinatus

Deltoid

Teres minor

Infraspinatus

Teres major

Rhomboid

Triceps

Latissimus dorsi

Sacrospinalis

Wrist extensors

Quadratus
lumborus

Gluteus
medius

Gluteus maximus

Piriformis

Gracilis

Hamstrings

Gastrocnemius

Posterior tibial

Soleus

BACK

the uptake of nutrients and leading to stiffness. Manipulating soft tissues relaxes them and increases blood flow so that oxygen and nutrients reach all of the tissues and waste such as lactic acid is removed. This repairs and strengthens muscles, easing pain and stiffness to increase the range of motion in joints, improve flexibility, and reduce the risk of injury. Easing muscular tension also improves alignment and, in turn, posture.

JOINTS AND TENDONS

Joints, the point where bones meet, give the skeleton flexibility. Tendons and ligaments are attached to joint capsules, such as at the shoulder and hips, or directly to bones, such as at the knee and elbow, allowing movement. Cartilage lies between bones, with synovial fluid cushioning them to prevent friction.

THE EFFECT OF MASSAGE

By stimulating circulation, massage nourishes the joints, promoting healing and preventing degenerative diseases. It also eases tension in tendons and ligaments to improve mobility and the range of motion.

FASCIA

The fibrous connective tissue known as fascia is a densely woven, continuous mesh covering each body structure. With healthy tissues, fascia is relaxed and wavy, able to stretch and move freely. After physical or mental trauma, scarring, inflammation, or repetitive actions, it thickens, losing pliability and tightening, which restricts movement and causes pain.

THE EFFECT OF MASSAGE

Deep tissue massage stretches the fascia, releasing adhesions that impede the flow of energy throughout the body.

NERVOUS SYSTEM

The nervous system is the control center of the body, sending and receiving signals to and from all parts of the body. Within the nervous system, there are divisions. The central nervous system (CNS) comprises the brain and the spinal cord. From the spinal cord, nerves branch out, forming the peripheral nervous system (PNS), which processes incoming sensory information.

The autonomic nervous system (ANS), which overlaps partly with the CNS and PNS, has its own nerve chains and regulates involuntary muscles, cardiac muscle, and certain glands, usually operating outside of our conscious control. There are further divisions within the autonomic nervous system. The sympathetic system is responsible for activating our "fight or flight," or stress response, while the parasympathetic division supports processes that conserve and restore energy during rest and recovery. The body is constantly working to balance these two responses in the nervous system.

THE EFFECT OF MASSAGE

During a massage, nerves in the skin are stimulated, acting on the CNS. This in turn activates the parasympathetic system, which is responsible for promoting restorative actions. As a result, the stress response is subdued and the body undergoes restorative processes, helping balance energy and encourage relaxation.

This state of relaxation helps optimize the functioning of body systems, helping these to work effectively. For example, when the circulatory system (see opposite) is supported and works smoothly, it nourishes tissues efficiently; also the liver and the lymphatic system (see p.22), unheeded by the effects of stress, metabolize and transport waste materials out of the body effectively.

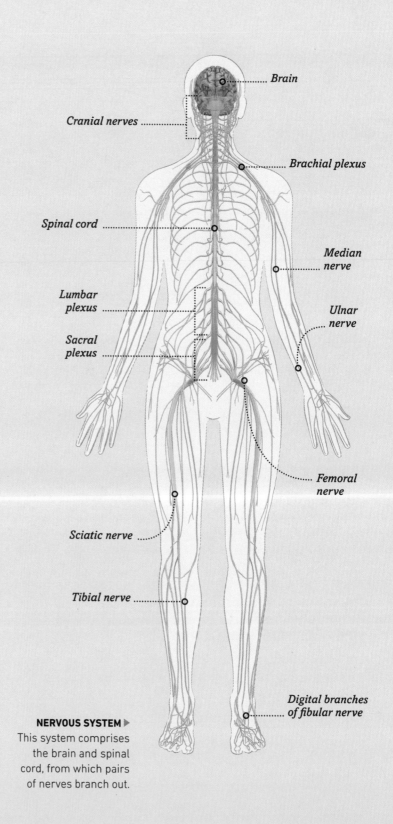

NERVOUS SYSTEM ▶
This system comprises the brain and spinal cord, from which pairs of nerves branch out.

Brain

Cranial nerves

Brachial plexus

Spinal cord

Median nerve

Lumbar plexus

Ulnar nerve

Sacral plexus

Femoral nerve

Sciatic nerve

Tibial nerve

Digital branches of fibular nerve

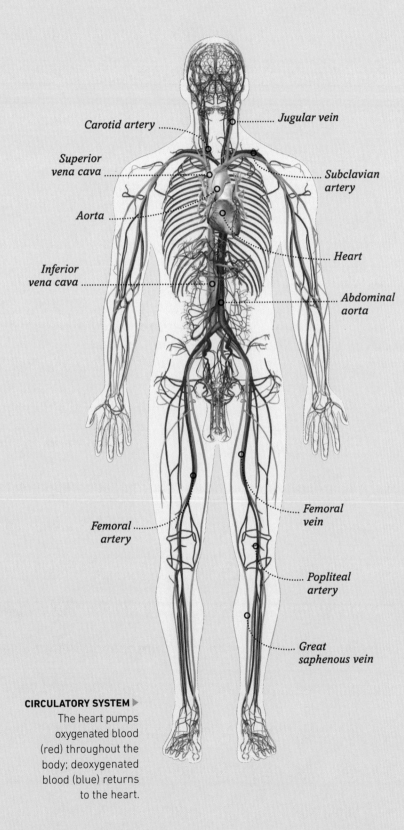

Carotid artery

Jugular vein

Superior
vena cava

Subclavian
artery

Aorta

Inferior
vena cava

Heart

Abdominal
aorta

Femoral
vein

Femoral
artery

Popliteal
artery

Great
saphenous vein

CIRCULATORY SYSTEM ▶
The heart pumps
oxygenated blood
(red) throughout the
body; deoxygenated
blood (blue) returns
to the heart.

CIRCULATORY SYSTEM
This is the body's transport hub, taking
oxygen and nutrients to tissues and cells
all over the body and picking up toxins and
waste products to expel.

THE EFFECT OF MASSAGE
Massage increases blood flow to an area.
When a part of the body is massaged, this
stimulates the circulation and blood rushes
to the area, replenishing it with nutrients and
oxygen and removing toxins. This in turn
stimulates the production of red and white
blood cells, increasing their numbers, and
encourages healing. A healthy circulation
also helps lower high blood pressure and
reduce the heart rate.

"Massaging a
particular part of
the body increases the
local circulation, bringing
blood to the area along
with nourishment
and oxygen."

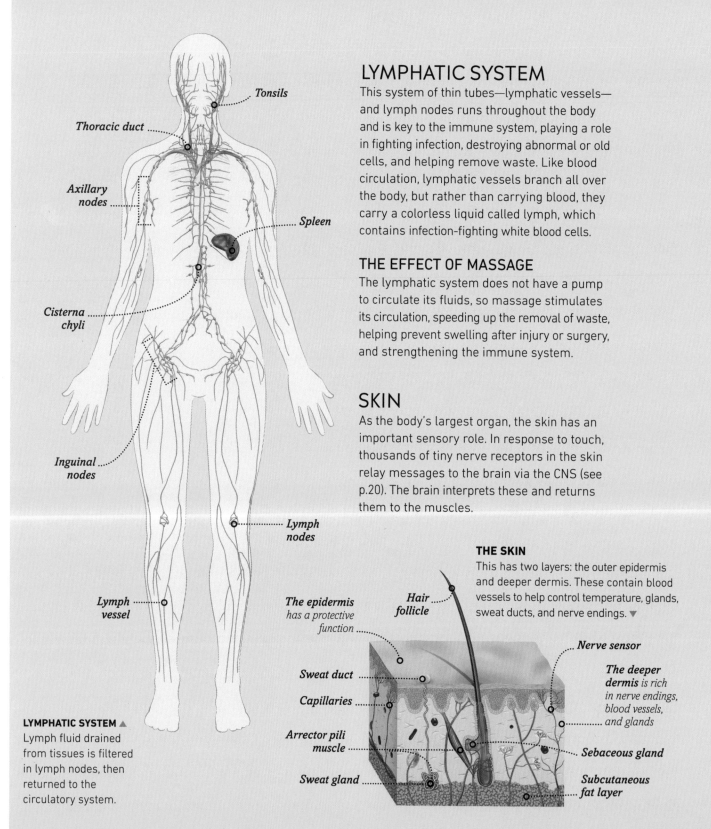

Tonsils

Thoracic duct

Axillary nodes

Spleen

Cisterna chyli

Inguinal nodes

Lymph nodes

Lymph vessel

LYMPHATIC SYSTEM

This system of thin tubes—lymphatic vessels—and lymph nodes runs throughout the body and is key to the immune system, playing a role in fighting infection, destroying abnormal or old cells, and helping remove waste. Like blood circulation, lymphatic vessels branch all over the body, but rather than carrying blood, they carry a colorless liquid called lymph, which contains infection-fighting white blood cells.

THE EFFECT OF MASSAGE

The lymphatic system does not have a pump to circulate its fluids, so massage stimulates its circulation, speeding up the removal of waste, helping prevent swelling after injury or surgery, and strengthening the immune system.

SKIN

As the body's largest organ, the skin has an important sensory role. In response to touch, thousands of tiny nerve receptors in the skin relay messages to the brain via the CNS (see p.20). The brain interprets these and returns them to the muscles.

THE SKIN

This has two layers: the outer epidermis and deeper dermis. These contain blood vessels to help control temperature, glands, sweat ducts, and nerve endings. ▼

The epidermis has a protective function

Hair follicle

Sweat duct

Capillaries

Arrector pili muscle

Sweat gland

Nerve sensor

The deeper dermis is rich in nerve endings, blood vessels, and glands

Sebaceous gland

Subcutaneous fat layer

LYMPHATIC SYSTEM ▲
Lymph fluid drained from tissues is filtered in lymph nodes, then returned to the circulatory system.

The skin comprises a superficial layer: the epidermis, and thicker connective tissue: the dermis. The tougher waterproof epidermis protects skin and underlying tissues by producing pigment, providing immune responses, and detecting touch sensations. The dermis, a fibrous layer of connective tissue, contains collagen and elastin proteins to give strength and elasticity. The dermis is also rich in tactile receptors, or microsensors, which are sensitive to touch.

THE EFFECT OF MASSAGE

Massage triggers the release of endorphins—our natural painkillers—sending messages to the nervous system to tell the body to relax. It also improves blood flow to the skin and stimulates sweat glands, both of which help remove toxins. Sebaceous glands in the dermis are also stimulated, aiding sebum production to lubricate skin. Also, by stimulating circulation, massage boosts the supply of nutrients to the skin via the blood, improving its texture and elasticity, and also supports the sloughing of dead cells, naturally exfoliating the skin. In addition, vegetable oils in massage provide their own nutrients and essential fatty acids that help nourish and feed the skin.

MAJOR ORGANS

Major organs such as the heart, lungs, liver, and stomach are controlled by the ANS (see p.20) and protected in the body by the ribcage. The organs are an integral part of the various body systems and are supplied with oxygen and nutrients from the circulatory system.

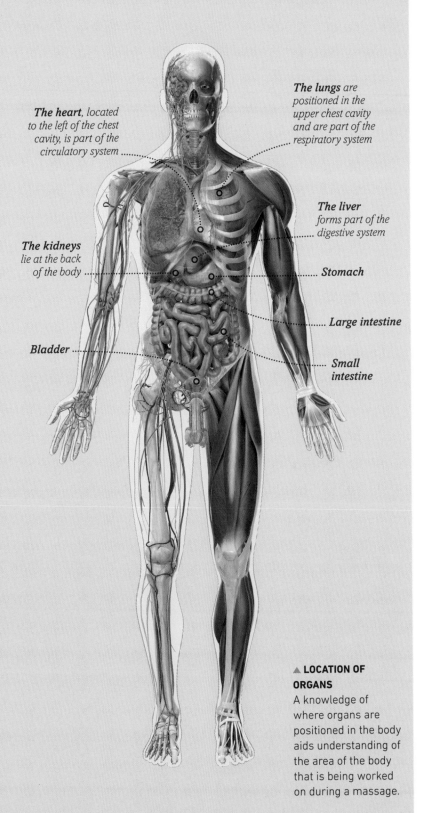

The heart, located to the left of the chest cavity, is part of the circulatory system

The lungs are positioned in the upper chest cavity and are part of the respiratory system

The liver forms part of the digestive system

The kidneys lie at the back of the body

Stomach

Large intestine

Bladder

Small intestine

▲ **LOCATION OF ORGANS**
A knowledge of where organs are positioned in the body aids understanding of the area of the body that is being worked on during a massage.

A GUIDE TO AROMATHERAPY

Aromatherapy is the therapeutic use of essential oils—the concentrated, fragrant, volatile essences extracted from plants—and has a long, established history in holistic healing, bringing harmony and balance to body and mind. Oils are selected for their unique properties to target specific complaints or simply increase well-being; used in massage blends, essential oils enhance the healing power of touch.

ROLE OF ESSENTIAL OILS

Each plant contains its own unique essential oil, made up of aromatic compounds thought to play a role in the plant's survival by warding off predators and attracting pollinators. When these essential oils are extracted from the plant, they contain these compounds in a concentrated form, capturing the essence and fragrance of the plant and harnessing its therapeutic benefits.

Essential oils are extracted from various parts of the plant, including berries, leaves, flowers, bark, roots, rind, and fruit. When you smell a rose or cut into a lemon, you inhale the essential oils. Oils are extracted using steam distillation and mechanical pressing.

QUALITY ASSURANCE

Always buy essential oils from a reputable source. Ideally, choose organic oils, free from synthetic fertilizers, pesticides, and herbicides.

components are dominant, often responsible for a distinct accent in the oil's aroma and determining its main therapeutic use; other components are minor, or trace elements within an oil. However, all of the components work synergistically; that is, the therapeutic power of the combined components is greater than that of one isolated component. So while it is possible to make synthetic fragrances by isolating a major component of an oil and combining it with other substances to make a comparable odor, the synthetic fragrances lack the complexity and magic of natural essential oils, not to mention their therapeutic effects.

WHAT'S IN ESSENTIAL OILS?

Each essential oil contains possibly hundreds of individual constituents, each contributing to its therapeutic value and fragrance. Certain

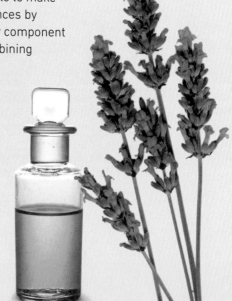

"When used in massage oil blends, essential oils enhance the therapeutic and holistic effects of the massage."

ESSENTIAL OILS IN MASSAGE

Our sense of smell is one of our most powerful, yet underused, senses. The body's response to smell is processed in the limbic brain, responsible for emotions and memories, which explains why certain smells can trigger strong emotional or physical responses. When we inhale an aroma, this triggers a response in the nervous system, influencing our mood, evoking emotions, and counteracting stress (or, if a smell memory is a negative one, provoking stress).

Aromatherapy is one of the most accessible and widely used natural remedies, and the holistic effects of essential oils are particularly relevant to conditions associated with modern-day living, such as stress, anxiety, and depression. Essential oils can be used to great effect in massage, where they are both inhaled, immediately stimulating the olfactory center in the forebrain, and absorbed through the skin, where they circulate around the body in the bloodstream, supporting and enhancing the relaxing, invigorating, and healing benefits of massage.

A massage practitioner will tailor their choice of essential oils to meet the specific needs of an individual so that the oil's inherent, unique properties can enhance the therapeutic and holistic benefits of the massage. For example, oils with warming, analgesic, and anti-inflammatory properties can be used to help soothe muscular aches and pains; those with revitalizing properties can support massage to stimulate sluggish circulation; and essential oils with calming and soothing effects can promote relaxation and good-quality sleep to help deal with concerns such as insomnia or stress. Because essential oils are highly concentrated substances they must always be diluted (see p.26) before applying them to the skin.

USING OILS SAFELY

Follow these guidelines when using concentrated essential oils.

- If an essential oil is spilled directly onto skin, dilute it with a base oil, then wash the area with soapy water.
- If an essential oil gets into the eyes, rinse the area with milk or plenty of cool water and seek medical advice.
- A patch test establishes sensitivity. A small amount of a diluted oil (at the percentage you want to use it, see p.27) is applied to the inner elbow. If no redness or irritation occurs within 24 hours, it can be used on a larger area. As it is not possible to test this during the duration of a massage treatment, establish if there is skin sensitivity at the start of the treatment and, if this is the case, use nonirritant oils (see p.28).
- Keep oils out of the reach of children.
- Some essential oils are flammable, so keep them away from candles, open flames, and any source of ignition.

BLENDING ESSENTIAL OILS

The highly concentrated nature of essential oils means that these natural extracts need to be diluted with a base, or carrier, oil before applying them to the skin (see chart, opposite). As well as diluting essential oils, base oils help disperse them, creating an oil blend that is easily spread over the skin.

BASE OILS

These have their own characteristics and therapeutic value, so being familiar with their properties will help you select appropriate oils for your massage needs. When choosing a base oil, consider factors such as the receiver's skin type and any sensitivities and whether a base oil has useful therapeutic benefits of its own for a particular complaint.

- Light oils such as almond, grapeseed, and coconut are good all-around oils, suitable for sensitive skins, but avoid nut-based oils if someone suffers from allergies. Almond is rich in skin-nourishing vitamin E and is slowly absorbed, so it is a popular choice for massage. Grapeseed is an odorless oil with a light, nongreasy finish and emollient properties, suitable for allergenic skin types. Coconut is semisolid but liquefies at body temperature, making it a light, easily absorbed oil that is moisturizing for dry skin.
- Heavier oils such as avocado, jojoba, and argan oil can be rich in nutrients and are particularly moisturizing. Avocado is high in enriching fatty acids, as well as vitamins A, D, and E, which can help condition rough skin. Jojoba oil is actually a wax that is liquid at room temperature; its waxy properties help trap moisture in the skin. Argan oil is high in fatty acids and vitamin E, making it a good choice for dry skin.
- Oils with extra therapeutic properties include macerated (plant-infused) oils such

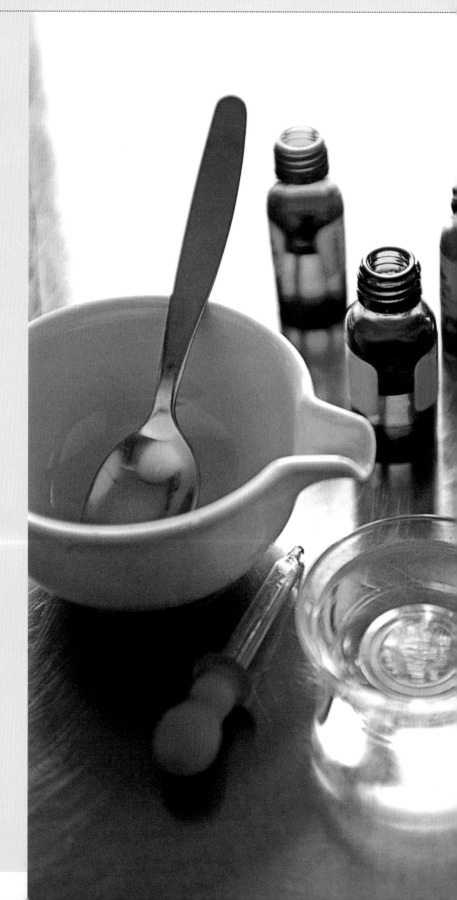

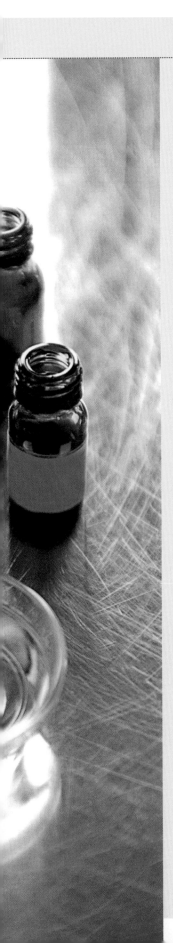

> *"As highly concentrated substances, essential oils need to be diluted in a base oil before being applied to the skin during a massage."*

as calendula, which soothes irritated skin; arnica, which has healing properties useful for sports injuries; and neem oil, which has antiseptic and anti-inflammatory properties.

GUIDE TO BLENDING OILS
Use about 2 tablespoons (30ml) of base oil for a full-body massage and 1 tablespoon (15ml) for the face or for local application. Follow this dilution guide of essential to base oils:
- 1 percent dilution for use on the face or with the elderly or children.
- 2.5 percent dilution for normal skin.
- 5 percent dilution for local application. The table below gives an example of dilutions for different massage uses and skin types.

STORING ESSENTIAL OILS
Essential oils need to be stored with care to preserve their delicate properties.
- Store oils in sterile glass or stainless-steel bottles with sealable lids. Dark-colored glass is best, as UV light can degrade the oil quality. Avoid plastic containers, as the oils will react with the plastic over time.
- Keep essential oils in a dark, cool place, away from heat and light.
- Make a note on the label of the date that the oil was opened.

DROPS OF ESSENTIAL OIL TO BASE PRODUCT			
Base oil	2 tsp/ 10ml	1 tbsp/ 15ml	2 tbsp/ 30ml
Essential oil for delicate skin or face blend	2 drops	3 drops	6 drops
Essential oil for whole-body blend	5 drops	7–8 drops (2.5% is 7½ drops)	15 drops
Local application	10 drops	15 drops	30 drops

CORE ESSENTIAL OILS FOR MASSAGE

When using essential oils in massage, you may want to begin with a core set of oils, then build on this as you grow familiar with different oils' properties and gain confidence blending. The 25 oils listed here have a range of therapeutic actions that can form the basis of your aromatherapy massage practice. This directory lists the characteristics of each oil together with recommended uses. The oils are safe used within the recommended dilutions (see p.27) unless stated otherwise. Do not use the oils if pregnant unless under the guidance of a qualified aromatherapist.

Anthemis nobilis
CHAMOMILE ROMAN
KEY ACTIONS: Relaxing, antispasmodic, anti-inflammatory.
USE FOR:
- **Mind** Insomnia, irritability, and anxiety.
- **Skin** Itchy, inflamed skin.
- **Musculoskeletal** Muscle aches, pains, inflammation.
- **Digestive** Cramps and spasms, IBS.
- **Women's health** Menstrual cramps, PMS.

Boswellia carterii
FRANKINCENSE
KEY ACTIONS: General tonic, uplifting.
USE FOR:
- **Mind** Anxiety, depression, chronic fatigue, exhaustion, stress, poor concentration.
- **Skin** Improves tone, facial use.
- **Musculoskeletal** Stress-related pains, fibromyalgia.
- **Respiratory** Chronic respiratory weakness, congestion, asthma.

Cananga odorata
YLANG YLANG
KEY ACTIONS: Uplifting, calming.
USE FOR:
- **Mind** Anxiety, depression, irritability, stress.
- **Skin** All types, acne, facial use.

- **Circulatory** Stress-related hypertension, palpitations.
- **Safety** Can cause headaches if sensitive to strong odors.

Cedrus atlantica
CEDARWOOD ATLAS
KEY ACTIONS: Balancing, warming, tonifying.
USE FOR:
- **Mind** Anxiety, depression, nervous tension, exhaustion.
- **Immunity** Lowered immunity, chronic fatigue.
- **Skin** Oily skin, acne.
- **Lymphatics** Sluggish lymphatics.
- **Respiratory** Chronic catarrh, asthma.

Citrus aurantium var. amara
NEROLI
KEY ACTIONS: Relaxing, refreshing, uplifting.
USE FOR:
- **Mind** Anxiety, depression, insomnia, stress, and tension.
- **Skin** All types, facial use, stretch marks and scars.
- **Digestive** Stress-related digestive issues, IBS.

Citrus bergamia
BERGAMOT
KEY ACTIONS: Balancing, uplifting.
USE FOR:
- **Mind** Mood swings, anxiety, depression.

- **Immunity** Aiding immunity.
- **Skin** Dry or oily skin.
- **Digestive** Indigestion, gas.
- **Safety** Use bergapten free to avoid problems with sunlight exposure.

Citrus limonum
LEMON
KEY ACTIONS: Cleansing, refreshing, uplifting.
USE FOR:
- **Mind** Depression, irritability, lethargy, tension headaches.
- **Immunity** Lowered immunity, convalescence.
- **Skin** Oily skin, acne.
- **Lymphatics:** Sluggish lymphatics.
- **Digestive** Sluggish digestion. **Safety** do not use above 2%—phototoxic (see p.244).

Citrus nobilis
MANDARIN
KEY ACTIONS: Soothing, antispasmodic.
USE FOR:
- **Mind** Anxiety, insomnia, irritability.
- **Skin** Oily skin, stretch marks.
- **Lymphatic system** Sluggish lymphatics
- **Digestive** Sluggish digestion, stress-related issues.

Cymbopogon martinii
PALMAROSA
KEY ACTIONS: Balancing, toning, cooling
USE FOR:
- **Mind** Anxiety, stress, irritability, exhaustion, tension headaches.
- **Skin** All types, acne, inflamed skin, facial use.
- **Circulatory** Palpitations.
- **Digestive** Indigestion, cramps and spasms.

Elettaria cardamomum
CARDAMOM
KEY ACTIONS: Uplifting, relaxing, warming, tonifying.
USE FOR:
- **Mind** Anxiety, depression,

nervous exhaustion, fatigue.
- **Immunity** Lowered immunity, chronic fatigue, convalescence.
- **Respiratory** Chronic respiratory congestion.
- **Digestive** Cramps and spasms, IBS, loss of appetite, sluggish digestion.

Eucalyptus globulus
EUCALYPTUS
KEY ACTIONS: Antimicrobial, antiseptic, stimulating.
USE FOR:
- **Mind** Fatigue, poor focus, sinus-related headaches.
- **Musculoskeletal** Muscle and joint pain, arthritis.
- **Respiratory** Respiratory tract infections, congestion.

Juniperus communis
JUNIPER
KEY ACTIONS: Warming, stimulating, detoxifying.
USE FOR:
- **Mind** Lethargy, tension.
- **Skin** Oily skin, acne.
- **Musculoskeletal** Muscle and joint pain, arthritis.
- **Circulatory** Poor circulation, cold extremities.
- **Lymphatics** Sluggish lymphatics, water retention.

Lavandula angustifolia
LAVENDER
KEY ACTIONS: Balancing, calming.
USE FOR:
- **Mind** Irritability, anxiety, depression, insomnia, shock, stress, nervous tension, headaches.
- **Skin** All skin types, acne, itchy and inflamed skin, scars and stretch marks.
- **Musculoskeletal** Muscle and joint pain, sciatica.
- **Circulatory** Stress-related hypertension.
- **Respiratory** Asthma, chest congestion, coughs.
- **Women's health** cramps, PMS, menopausal symptoms.

Litsea cubeba
MAY CHANG
KEY ACTIONS: Relaxing, tonifying, uplifting.
USE FOR:
- **Mind** Depression, fatigue, lethargy.
- **Immunity** Lowered immunity, chronic fatigue.
- **Skin** Oily skin, acne.
- **Musculoskeletal** Stress-related muscle pains, fibromyalgia.
- **Circulatory** Stress-related palpitations.
- **Respiratory** Asthma.
- **Digestive** Indigestion, cramps and spasms.
- **Safety** Do not use above 2%, with children or sensitive skin. Do patch test.

Mentha piperita
PEPPERMINT
KEY ACTIONS: Cools and then warms, refreshing, stimulating.
USE FOR:
- **Mind** Fatigue, poor focus, sinus-related headaches.
- **Musculoskeletal** Muscle and joint pain, arthritis, sprains and strains.
- **Circulatory** Poor circulation.
- **Respiratory** Upper and lower tract infections, congestion.
- **Digestive** Cramps, spasms, IBS, sluggish digestion.
- **Safety** Do not use over 1% with sensitive skin.

Origanum marjorana
• SWEET MARJORAM
KEY ACTIONS: Analgesic, strengthening, relaxing.
USE FOR:
- **Mind** Anxiety, insomnia, exhaustion, tension headaches.
- **Musculoskeletal** Muscle and joint pain, fibromyalgia.
- **Circulatory** Stress-related palpitations.
- **Respiratory** Chest congestion, asthma.
- **Digestive** Indigestion, cramps and spasms.

Pelargonium graveolens
GERANIUM
KEY ACTIONS: Cooling, moistening, balancing.
USE FOR:
- **Mind** Mood swings, anxiety, depression.
- **Skin** Balancing for all skin types, facial use with acne.
- **Digestive** Stress-related digestive complaints.
- **Women's health** PMS and menopausal symptoms.

Pinus sylvestris
PINE
KEY ACTIONS: Antimicrobial, energizing, warming.
USE FOR:
- **Mind** Nervous exhaustion, sciatica.
- **Musculoskeletal** Muscle and joint pain, arthritis, sprains and strains.
- **Circulatory** Poor circulation, cold extremities.
- **Respiratory** Acute infections.
- **Safety** Below 2% with sensitive skin.

Piper nigrum
BLACK PEPPER
KEY ACTIONS: Warming, stimulating, energizing.
USE FOR:
- **Mind** Exhaustion, sciatica.
- **Immunity** Lowered immunity, convalescence.
- **Musculoskeletal** Muscle and joint pain, arthritis.
- **Circulatory** Poor circulation, cold extremities.
- **Respiratory** Coughs, chest congestion.
- **Safety** Not for facial use.

Pogostemon cablin
PATCHOULI
KEY ACTIONS: Balancing, strengthening.
USE FOR:
- **Mind** Anxiety, nervous exhaustion, stress.
- **Immunity** Weak immunity.
- **Skin** Oily skin, acne, scars, stretch marks.

- **Lymphatic system** Sluggish lymphatics.
- **Digestion** Sluggish digestion, stress-related digestive issues, IBS.

Rosa damascena
ROSE
KEY ACTIONS: Relaxing, cooling, tonifying.
USE FOR:
- **Mind** Anxiety, depression, stress.
- **Skin** Dry, mature, sensitive, or inflamed skin, facial use.
- **Digestive** Sluggish digestion, especially stress-related.
- **Women's health** PMS and menopausal symptoms.

Rosmarinus officinalis
ROSEMARY
KEY ACTIONS: Stimulating, warming, analgesic.
USE FOR:
- **Mind** Lethargy, poor focus, depression, headaches.
- **Musculoskeletal** Muscle and joint pain, arthritis.
- **Circulatory** Poor circulation, cold extremities.
- **Digestion** Sluggish digestion, cramps, spasms.
- **Women's health** Painful menstrual cramps.
  Safety Caution with epilepsy if not from a reputable source.

Thymus vulgaris CT linalool
THYME LINALOOL
KEY ACTIONS: Warming, antimicrobial, tonifying.
USE FOR:
- **Mind** Exhaustion, stress, tension, depression.
- **Immunity** Lowered immunity, chronic fatigue, convalescence.
- **Musculoskeletal** Muscle and joint pain, arthritis, strains and sprains, muscle weakness, loss of tone.
- **Respiratory** Infections and chronic congestion.
- **Digestive** cramps and spasms, IBS, loss of

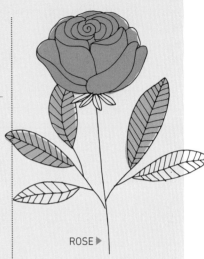

ROSE ▶

appetite, sluggish digestion.
- **Safety** Use reputable source.

Vetiveria zizanoides
VETIVER
KEY ACTIONS: Sedating, strengthening, warming.
USE FOR:
- **Mind** Anxiety, insomnia, exhaustion.
- **Skin** All types, acne.
- **Musculoskeletal** Muscle and joint pain, sprains and strains, arthritis.
- **Circulatory** Poor circulation.
- **Lymphatics** Sluggish lymphatics.

Zingiber officinale
GINGER
KEY ACTIONS: Warming, stimulating.
USE FOR:
- **Mind** Exhaustion, chronic fatigue.
- **Musculoskeletal** Muscle and joint pain, arthritis.
- **Circulatory** Poor circulation, cold extremities.
- **Digestive** Cramps and spasms, indigestion.
- **Women's health** Painful periods.

BEING PREPARED

Aside from honing your massage techniques, there are other important ways to prepare for and develop your practice. Being properly equipped and spending some time on your mental and physical preparation (see pp.32–35) will ensure that when it comes to the actual massage, you will be able to place your focus solely on the receiver, knowing that all of the accompanying elements are in place to allow treatments to run as smoothly as possible.

TOOLS OF THE TRADE

Whether in a practice, a dedicated space in your home, or at the receiver's home, a massage environment should be welcoming, clean, and calm. In addition, being properly equipped will ensure the comfort of both you and the receiver, allowing you both to relax.

ESSENTIALS

A massage table or comfortable, supportive surface is key. A dedicated massage bed is ideal. For occasional massage, a well-padded, supportive floor-based futon can be used. Most beds are too soft for a massage and at an awkward height that puts pressure on the back. When choosing a massage table, look for the main features (see right) and make sure it is stable. Some tables state a weight limit, so check if this suits your needs. If you need to travel, a lighter, portable table is ideal.

Clean towels and table covers are a must. A cover offers hygiene, while towels ensure comfort, warmth, and privacy and provide a safe boundary between practitioner and receiver. You will need the following:
• A protective cover, clean cotton sheet, or

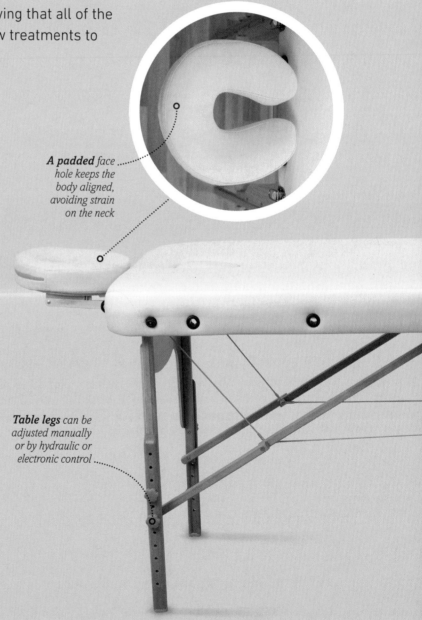

A padded face hole keeps the body aligned, avoiding strain on the neck

Table legs can be adjusted manually or by hydraulic or electronic control

large towels to cover the table.

- A disposable paper cover can be used on top of the couch cover or towels; otherwise, launder towels and cover after each client.
- Two large towels to cover the receiver (see p.81). Only one part of the body at a time—the part about to be treated—is uncovered.
- Extra towels to roll up or fold for support and comfort. These can be placed under the ankles when the receiver is face down (prone); under the knees when face up (supine) to alleviate pressure on the hips and relax the lower back and stomach; and under the head for support.

Lubricants such as oils, lotions, waxes, and powders help the hands to glide.

- Vegetable oils, such as grapeseed and sweet almond, are commonly

A table that can be raised at the head to semi-upright allows you to adapt the massage to a person's needs

used (see p.26). These are easily absorbed, skin-nourishing, and can be stored in a pump bottle for quick, hygienic access. They also warm up quickly.

- Waxes are firmer and provide more grip if desired. They are often combined with oils for a semisolid texture.
- Powders may be used in reflexology, providing a nonslippery medium.

EXTRAS

In addition to the core items above, you may also want to include the following in your massage practice:

Pillows to enhance comfort and offer additional support. They can be used in place of rolled towels under the ankles and knees.

A chair for a head and shoulder massage or for a back massage with the receiver sitting astride it if possible, using cushions as comfortable padding if needed.

Essential oils to blend with base oils to enhance the massage (see pp.24–29).

Meditative music, if welcome, to create a relaxing, peaceful environment and/or to block out background noise.

Unscented candles may be used to create an inviting environment.

◀ **COMFORT AND CARE**
Look for a well-cushioned table with a wipe-clean surface.

PRACTICAL AND PHYSICAL PREPARATION

As well as ensuring you have all the right equipment in place (see pp.30–31), consider practicalities, such as room temperature and what you are wearing. During the massage, your posture, balance, and how you move around is key, both for facilitating the massage and to ensure that you don't injure yourself. Check the list below to make sure you are prepped and take some time to practice the postures, opposite.

BEFORE YOU START

A comfortable, warm, peaceful environment will help promote a relaxed atmosphere for both you and the receiver. Make sure that you are both suitably prepared and that any possible distractions have been removed.

- Keep the room warm enough for the receiver when he or she is undressed, but not so warm that it is unbearable for you. Massage should be as relaxing and therapeutic to give as it is to receive.
- Turn your phones off and, ideally, make sure that these are out of sight.
- Don't wear jewelry and ask the receiver to remove theirs. Rings, watches, and bracelets could catch on skin and potentially scratch one of you, while noisy jewelry can be a distraction.
- Ask the receiver to remove glasses or, if massaging the face, their contact lenses.
- Keep your nails short so they can't dig into the receiver's skin.
- Wear comfortable, nonrestrictive clothing. Cotton is preferable to synthetic fibers to stop you getting sweaty and overheated.
- Adjust the table to suit your height. Stand straight with your hands at your sides and make a fist. The table should be level with your first set of knuckles. You may need to lower the table for deeper tissue work.

- Have at hand previous notes, a pen, any relevant reference material, and have a clock in view.

MASSAGE POSTURE

Body mechanics and posture are extremely important for massage therapists to ensure balance and fluid movement and to avoid injury. Depth of stroke should come from using body weight and should be driven by the lower limbs, not by tensing or pushing from the hands, arms, or shoulders.

When standing, both feet should be in contact with the floor, the back should be straight, the shoulders relaxed down, and the chest open. Avoid overstretching, always face in the direction of the strokes, and don't stay in one position for too long.

Adopt the positions, opposite, to suit different techniques. Work on the head can also be done while seated, with the legs spread wide and feet flat on the floor.

APPLYING OILS

Just a small amount of oil is needed for a massage. Too much oil can be slippery and prevent good control, while too little can irritate skin by pulling the hairs. Generally, long effleurage strokes (see p.40) require more oil to allow the hands to glide. Always oil your hands rather than placing oil straight on the body, following the guide below:

- Apply a small amount of oil to the palm of one hand. Rub your hands together to warm the oil before using it.

- Carry on adding small amounts of oil as needed. To avoid breaking contact when reapplying oil, rest one cupped hand, palm up, on the back. Squeeze a little oil into the

hand, returning the bottle to a safe, reachable place. Lay the other palm on the cupped one and gently spread the oil between them. Turn both hands over to resume strokes. Done properly, the receiver may not even notice.

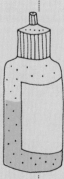

TRAPEZIUS STRETCH

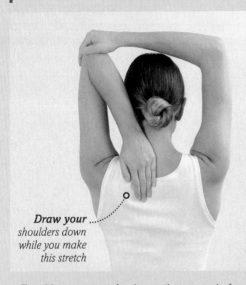

Draw your shoulders down while you make this stretch

▲ **Try this arm stretch**, alternating arms, before you start to open up the chest and stretch the trapezius to release tension and improve mobility.

SIDEWAYS LUNGE

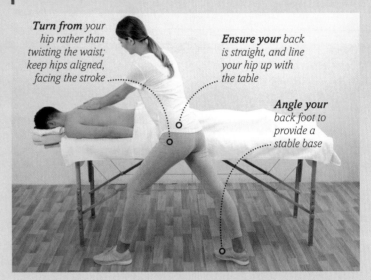

Turn from your hip rather than twisting the waist; keep hips aligned, facing the stroke

Ensure your back is straight, and line your hip up with the table

Angle your back foot to provide a stable base

▲ **Use this position** for gliding effleurage strokes (see p.40). Step back with the leg closest to the table, then bend your front knee to lunge. Lunge back and forth to work up and down the body.

KNEELING STANCE

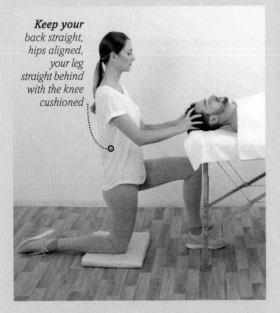

Keep your back straight, hips aligned, your leg straight behind with the knee cushioned

▲ **A kneeling stance** at the top of the table can be used for head work. From kneeling, step a leg in to 90 degrees, keeping the knee aligned with the foot.

SQUATTING SIDE ON

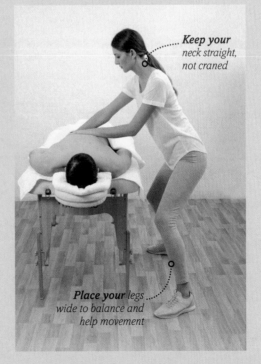

Keep your neck straight, not craned

Place your legs wide to balance and help movement

◀ **Facing the table** and adopting a squatting position allows you to work across to the opposite side of the body, which is useful for deeper petrissage work (see p.56). Align your pelvis with the table and squat so that your arms can work across the body without flexing the wrists. Sway your legs side to side to work up and down an area.

MENTAL PREPARATION

In addition to physical and practical preparation (see pp.32–33), preparing yourself mentally—"getting into the zone"—is an essential part of the practice. Being grounded, calm, and focused will allow you to give the massage your undivided attention and in turn help the receiver to let go and completely relax.

Before you begin a massage, your mind needs to feel calm and free from distractions. Different techniques and lifestyle practices can help you master the stillness and focus you need to optimize your practice.

GIVE YOURSELF ENOUGH TIME

Building in sufficient time so you can take stock before a session will ensure that you don't feel rushed and out of sync and that you are in a calm state of mind. Create a schedule that gives you a quiet interval between appointments so you have time to carry out any relaxation or stretching techniques (see opposite and p.33) if you wish to do so; too many back-to-back appointments should be avoided.

If you need to travel to a practice or client, arrive early so that you don't feel rushed and you have time to prepare—checking that the room is clean and warm and that everything you need is at hand. Making sure that the environment is restful, welcoming, and comfortable will be mentally soothing for both you and the receiver.

STAYING GROUNDED

As a massage therapist, your calm demeanor is an important element. Being grounded and feeling mentally "still" will set the receiver at ease from the outset, helping him or her to step back from the emotional state they arrived in. Maintaining this stillness throughout the massage will enhance the feeling of relaxation. The ability to stay grounded will also help you not to take on

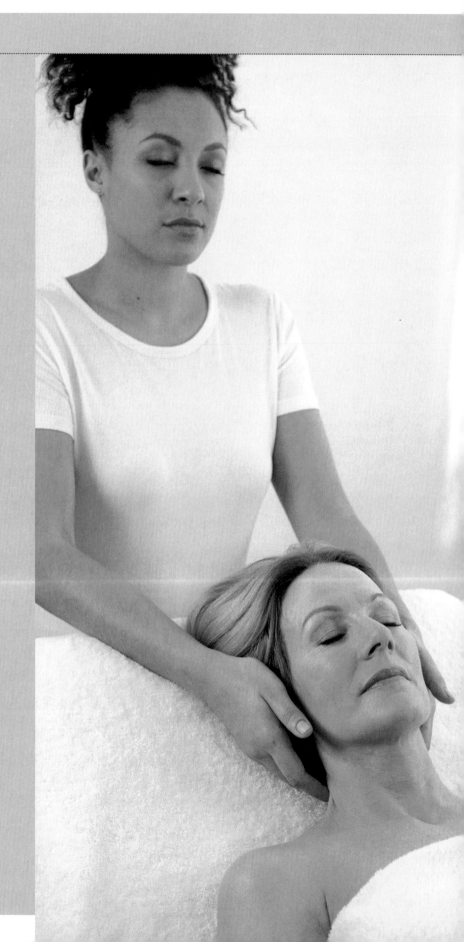

the emotions of the receiver or carry these through the day into other appointments. You may want to try some of the following techniques and practices:

- Practice meditative breathing exercises (see below) to calm the mind. Breathe from the diaphragm and focus on your breath, letting go of any intrusive thoughts. Breathing into any areas of tension also helps you to release physical stress. As you relax with your breaths, you will feel tension ebb away.
- Try the following yoga breathing exercise.
1 Sit in a comfortable position, close your eyes, and breathe quietly through your nostrils, observing the sound of your breath as you breathe in and out.
2 After a minute or so, lengthen your inhalation slightly, followed by a usual exhalation. Do this for five breaths, then breathe normally for a few breaths.
3 Next, lengthen your exhalation, followed by a normal inhalation, for five breaths.
4 Return to normal breathing once more, then finally lengthen both inhalation and exhalation for five breaths before returning to normal breathing to end the exercise.
- Try visualizations to calm your mind. Imagine a warm light enveloping your body to help you relax. Or imagine that your feet have roots deep in the ground while your spine and neck float up like the top of a tree to help you embody spaciousness and feel grounded. Or try your own visualizations to help you feel present, calm, and responsive.
- Listen to calming, meditative music to prepare and focus before a treatment. You may wish to play this throughout a

treatment if the receiver is happy for you to do so, which can also help relax them and ensure that he or she doesn't feel the need to make conversation.

LOOKING AFTER YOURSELF

Massage can be physically and emotionally demanding, so to ensure that you feel mentally resilient and able to relax during the treatment, you need to look after yourself. Staying fit and agile, eating healthily, avoiding alcohol, and getting sufficient sleep will all enhance your ability to massage. Part of looking after yourself is learning how to manage everyday stress. Try to make time for activities that energize, revitalize, and, in turn, relax you, such as being out in nature. Try to limit screen time, too, perhaps allocating a set time of the day to catch up on news or social media. Also be aware of your body's natural rhythms and try to schedule appointments for when your energy levels are optimal.

GIVING AND RECEIVING

Massage is a reciprocal practice. Your deeply relaxed state influences a treatment; likewise, sensing the receiver's relaxation helps ground you.

STARTING THE SESSION

Starting the session off with a friendly yet professional conversation will help build a relationship based on trust. Introduce yourself and ask how the receiver is feeling and why they have booked a treatment. This friendly introduction and inquiry, followed by a discussion of your treatment plan (see pp.176–177), will relax both you and the receiver. Tell the receiver to give you feedback if they wish, letting you know where pressure is too soft or hard and any areas that need more attention.

A SAFE PRACTICE

Massage should always be a positive and therapeutic experience for both giver and receiver. To ensure that this is the case, it's essential to be aware of contraindications that mean massage should be avoided. Also think about how you can maintain professional boundaries between yourself and the receiver to make sure that you both feel completely comfortable and safe.

CONTRAINDICATIONS

Massage should be avoided where it could aggravate a complaint or impact health. Also, never try to diagnose a health problem; instead, advise the recipient to visit a qualified medical practitioner. Avoid massage in these situations:

- If either you or the receiver has a fever or is in pain, or if you feel unwell or very tired.
- If someone has thrombosis.
- With open wounds, broken bones, bruises, joint dislocation, or soft tissue ruptures.
- If you have broken or damaged skin (even minor damage) on your hands or forearms.
- On local areas where the receiver has a possibly contagious condition, such as athlete's foot, a wart, or a cold sore.
- If there are areas of major inflammation with heat, redness, or a burn.
- Where there is swelling caused by arthritis.
- If someone has epilepsy—refer for medical advice before a massage.
- You may wish to avoid massage until the second trimester of pregnancy, when the risk of miscarriage is reduced.
- Avoid aromatherapy on breastfeeding women unless supervised by a professional.
- If someone is under the influence of alcohol or recreational drugs.

PERSONAL PRESENTATION
Maintaining personal hygiene is crucial; keep nails neatly trimmed and hands scrupulously clean.▼

MASSAGE HYGIENE

A crucial part of providing a safe treatment is ensuring hygiene.

- Be clean and presentable. Wash your hands before and after a treatment and before touching the face.
- Tie long hair back and, if you are likely to sweat, wear a head band to create a barrier.
- Keep your nails short.
- Avoid wearing strong-smelling perfume or cologne.
- Make sure the towels do not touch the floor at any point before or during a treatment.

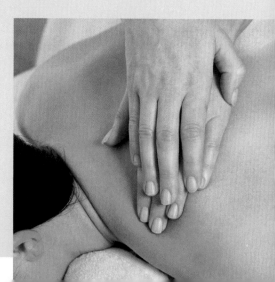

THINKING ABOUT BOUNDARIES

Establishing boundaries between yourself and the receiver helps avoid confusion and ensure a safe practice. Some practices are down to personal choice—for example, how much you talk to each other, what you wear, the products you use, whether to exchange gifts, and how you communicate when arranging a massage. There are also physical, emotional, and social boundaries to be aware of.

PHYSICAL BOUNDARIES

Setting physical boundaries is very important. The receiver is in a vulnerable position during a treatment, so proceeding with care and sensitivity ensures trust. Using towels correctly, covering the body and uncovering just the part you need access to, maintains the modesty of the receiver and helps them to feel secure and comfortable.

Tell the receiver to let you know if they are not happy with anything and explain what you are going to do before moving a towel. Never expose the genitals, breasts, or buttocks and adapt techniques around the upper thigh to avoid the genital area. Tell the receiver if you need to move the towel lower to work on the gluteals.

Just as the practitioner should not touch the receiver inappropriately, the receiver also should not touch the therapist inappropriately. If this happens, make it clear that this behavior is undesired and, if necessary, end the session and do not reschedule the person.

EMOTIONAL BOUNDARIES

Emotional boundaries help keep massage relationships on a professional footing. If a receiver tries to make the relationship personal, this is known as transference. This may be happening if he or she suggests a meal, contacts you outside working hours, asks for a reduced price, or brings you gifts. Being aware of this means you can steer the relationship back to a professional level.

Countertransference is when the therapist offloads problems or finds it hard to separate personal feelings from a therapeutic relationship. A therapist may think excessively about someone after a treatment or believe that they can remove all of their pain. If this occurs, it's important to check these feelings. Practitioners may find that committing to periodic professional supervision or mentoring will help maintain and refine their own best practice.

CARE AND SENSITIVITY

Properly applied, massage is unlikely to cause an adverse reaction, but too much pressure or over-treating an area could cause inflammation.

SOCIAL BOUNDARIES

These are most commonly crossed. Talking is a normal interaction, but as a therapist, you should control the urge to ask about work, home life, or vacations. Likewise, if the receiver drifts toward conversation, this may be a sign of nervousness, so you need to bring the receiver back to a relaxing, therapeutic environment where silence is comfortable and the focus is on the massage only.

If someone is a colleague, family member, or acquaintance, it can be hard to maintain boundaries. You may feel obliged to offer a discount or greater flexibility, which can be demotivating. You may wish to limit or avoid such relationships, perhaps recommending a fellow therapist to avoid any awkwardness.

BASIC TECHNIQUES

The core set of techniques that make up Swedish massage (see p.110) form the foundation of massage practice in the West. These techniques make up the practitioner's toolkit and are combined to create the ebb and flow of a massage, allowing the practitioner or giver to build pressure gradually. The techniques are also integrated into many massage specialties so that tissues can be softened and relaxed before applying more targeted pressure. Throughout a treatment, effleurage and petrissage soften the tissues and promote deep relaxation; lively percussions stimulate and wake the body up; and vibrations, static pressures, and passive movements loosen areas of resistance.

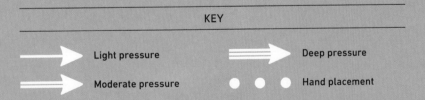

KEY

Light pressure

Moderate pressure

Deep pressure

Hand placement

BASIC TECHNIQUES
EFFLEURAGE STROKES

These flowing, rhythmic, smooth strokes form the basis of massage. As introductory strokes, they connect giver and receiver, beginning a dialogue through touch; practically, they spread oil so you can work without dragging the skin and they warm the tissues, boosting circulation. Effleurage is akin to a melody that you return to between other strokes, connecting different strokes together, as well as the receiver to their body. Each stroke should be done at least three times in a continuous action. The speed can vary, but the deeper you go, the more slowly you should work to sense if you are going too deeply and causing contraction rather than release. Generally, strokes are deeper toward the heart and lighter gliding back.

FAN STROKE

WHEN TO USE	GOOD FOR	PRESSURE
Start of massage	**Applying oil and warming tissues**	**Mostly moderate to deep**

The T-shaped fan stroke is an oil-spreading stroke done on the back either from the base of the spine, as shown, or from the top of the back, with the T shape opening out across the sacrum. The stroke can be done in stages, making mini-fans or fountains, as shown here, or, if oil has already been applied, you can make one large fan over the back. As you repeat the stroke, tissues gradually warm up and relax, allowing you to deepen the pressure.

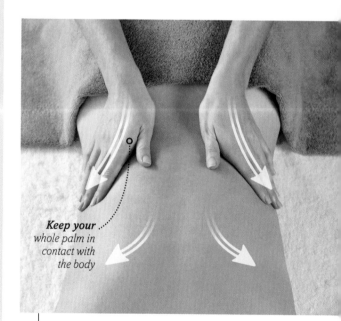

Keep your whole palm in contact with the body

 Lean in, using the weight of your body to help apply pressure, and fan your hands out in small fountainlike actions. Repeat this pattern up the back, reapplying oil at any point if needed (see p.32).

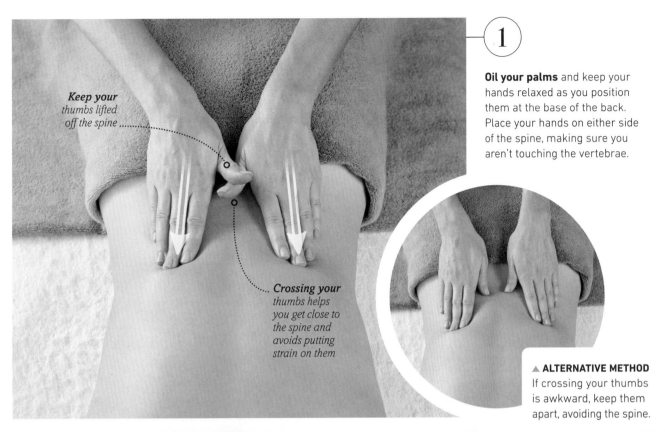

Keep your thumbs lifted off the spine ......

Crossing your thumbs helps you get close to the spine and avoids putting strain on them

(1)

Oil your palms and keep your hands relaxed as you position them at the base of the back. Place your hands on either side of the spine, making sure you aren't touching the vertebrae.

▲ **ALTERNATIVE METHOD**
If crossing your thumbs is awkward, keep them apart, avoiding the spine.

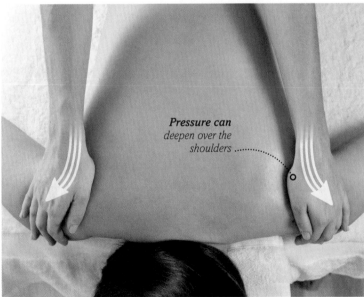

Pressure can deepen over the shoulders ......

(3) **As you reach** the shoulders, fan out your hands simultaneously in a large T shape, keeping your fingers relaxed and increasing the pressure as you lean into the stroke.

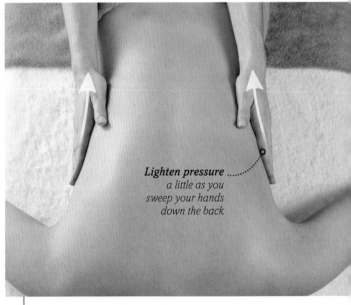

Lighten pressure a little as you sweep your hands down the back

(4) **Slide your hands** around to the sides of the ribcage and sweep back down the entire length of the back, making sure that your hands don't lose contact with the back at any point as you prepare to repeat the stroke.

THOUSAND HANDS

WHEN TO USE
Start of massage
or if skin dries

GOOD FOR
Spreading oil;
warming hands

PRESSURE
Light to
moderate

This smooth, flowing action is an oil-spreading technique done over large surface areas such as the back or limbs. As well as oiling the skin, it also warms your hands and introduces touch. As your hands alternate in small, gliding strokes, one hand always in contact, the receiver has the sensation of lots of hands working on the body.

OVER THE SKIN

Place the whole palm of one hand on the body. Glide your hand up the body, then lift your hand and begin a new stroke with your other hand, alternating hands constantly to ensure that one hand is always in contact with the body.

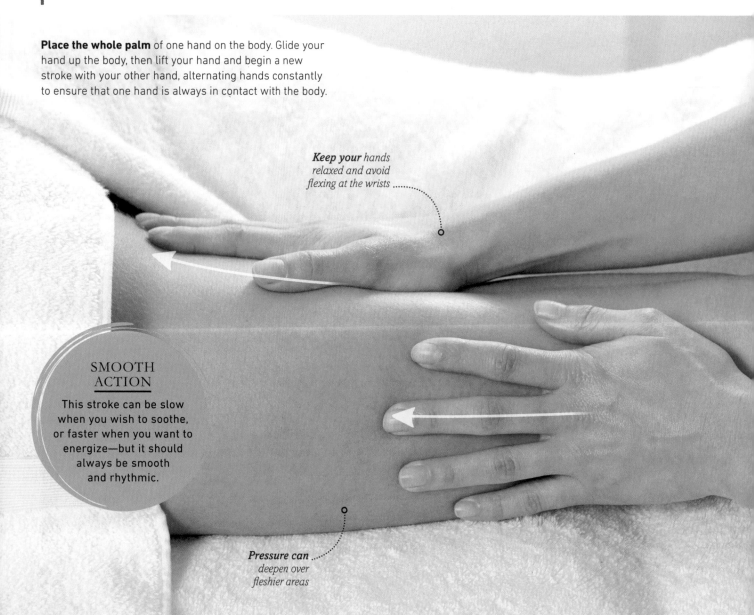

Keep your hands relaxed and avoid flexing at the wrists

SMOOTH ACTION

This stroke can be slow when you wish to soothe, or faster when you want to energize—but it should always be smooth and rhythmic.

Pressure can deepen over fleshier areas

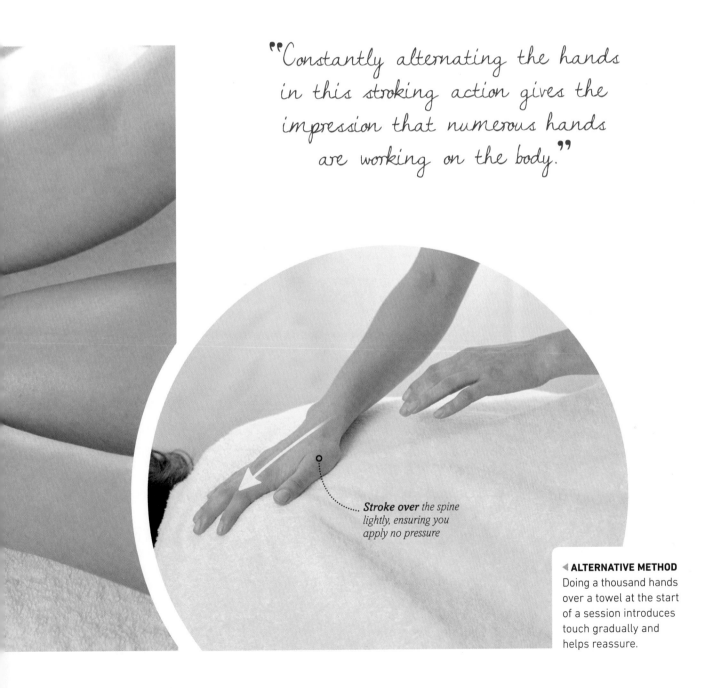

"Constantly alternating the hands in this stroking action gives the impression that numerous hands are working on the body."

Stroke over the spine lightly, ensuring you apply no pressure

◀ **ALTERNATIVE METHOD**
Doing a thousand hands over a towel at the start of a session introduces touch gradually and helps reassure.

SLIDE AND GLIDE STROKES

WHEN TO USE
At the start of work to an area

GOOD FOR
Applying oil; warming tissues

PRESSURE
Build to moderate with repetitions

These fluid, oil-applying strokes, used at the start of massage to an area or if the skin dries out, also gently stretch and warm the underlying tissues to oxygenate the area and help you sense points of tension. Lightly oil your hands, then repeat a stroke at least three times on each area, working progressively deeper each time.

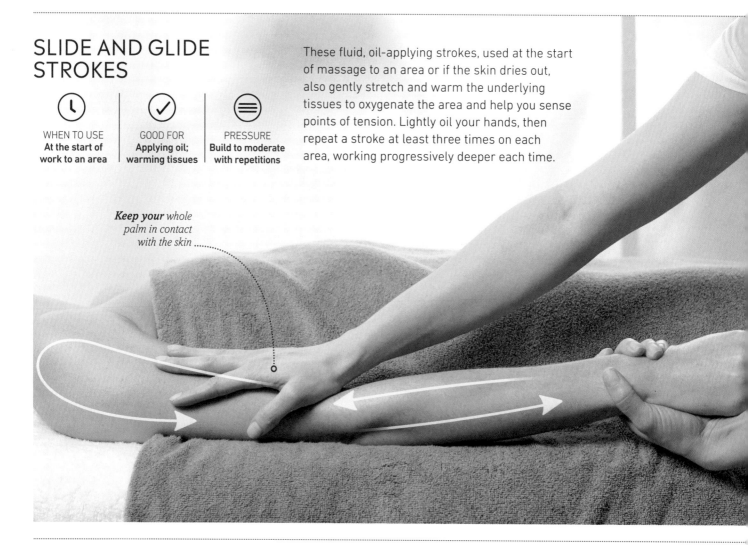

Keep your whole *palm in contact with the skin*

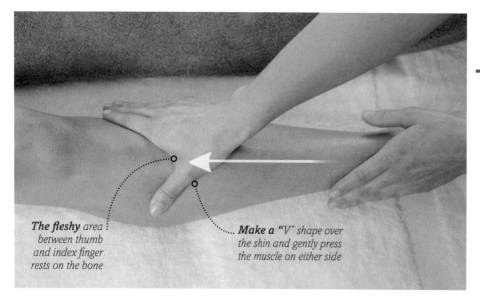

The fleshy area *between thumb and index finger rests on the bone*

Make a "V" shape over the shin and gently press the muscle on either side

— OVER THE SHIN BONE

◄ **This technique,** called "dragon's mouth," cups your hand over the shin bone. It is unique to the shin, as it allows you to work on the lower limb without pressing on the bone, while the leg shape here prevents your thumb joint overextending. Glide up to the knee, then sweep back down the calf side as your other hand starts a new stroke.

OVER THE CHEST AND SHOULDERS

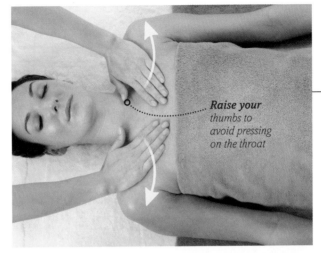

Raise your thumbs to avoid pressing on the throat

1

Standing behind the head, knees slightly bent, place your palms on either side of the chest, being careful with this delicate area. Fan your hands out to cup the shoulders.

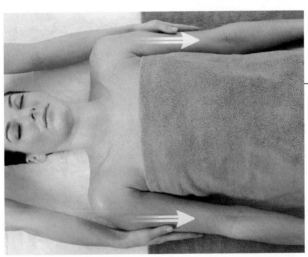

2

Keeping the whole of your palms in contact with the body, sweep down the shoulders and tops of the arms, using your body weight to lean in as you deepen pressure over this fleshier area.

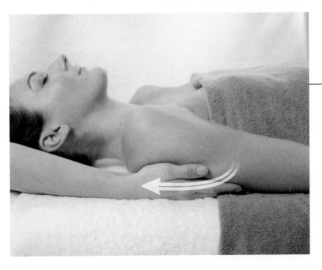

3

Curve your palms under the arms and sweep back up, taking your hands right under the shoulders. Repeat the steps several times in a continuous action, increasing the pressure in step 2 each time.

ALONG THE ARM

◀ **Gently hold the wrist** to stabilize and slightly stretch the arm while you sweep up the length of the arm with your other hand. Circle the shoulder and glide back down in an elongated "O" shape. Swap hands and repeat several times in a fluid, rhythmic movement. Turn the arm to repeat on the inner arm.

SENSE OF TOUCH

These introductory strokes engage communication between the nerves and muscles and help the receiver get a sense of your touch.

CIRCLE STROKES

WHEN TO USE
After initial
warm-up strokes

GOOD FOR
Circulation boost;
tension release

PRESSURE
Moderate
to deep

Working the tissues in a circular motion helps to warm them, boosting circulation to an area, and also releases stickiness in the superficial fascia that can cause tension and pain. Circle strokes are helpful in areas where tension is typically held, such as the shoulders and back, or for releasing tightness in muscly areas such as the thighs. Pressure can vary from moderate to deep; ensure that you slow the stroke the deeper you go.

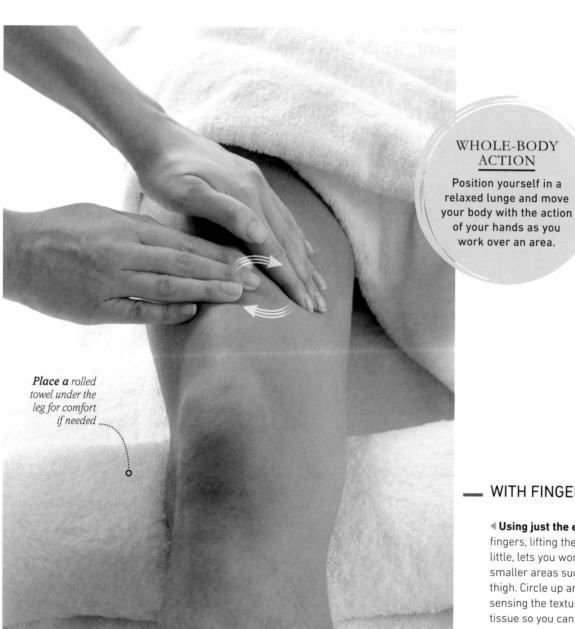

WHOLE-BODY ACTION

Position yourself in a relaxed lunge and move your body with the action of your hands as you work over an area.

Place a rolled towel under the leg for comfort if needed

WITH FINGERS

◄ **Using just the ends** of the fingers, lifting the palm a little, lets you work into smaller areas such as the thigh. Circle up and down, sensing the texture of the tissue so you can detect areas of tightness—for example, in the quadriceps.

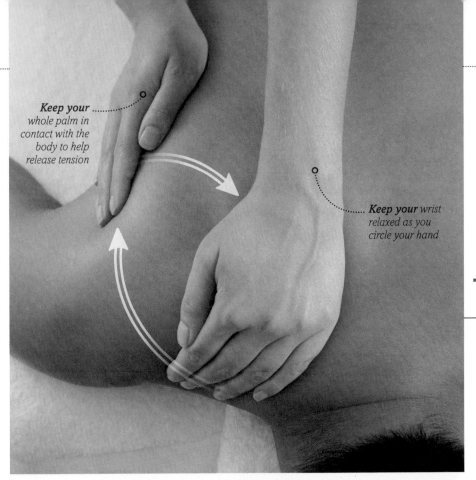

Keep your whole palm in contact with the body to help release tension

Keep your wrist relaxed as you circle your hand

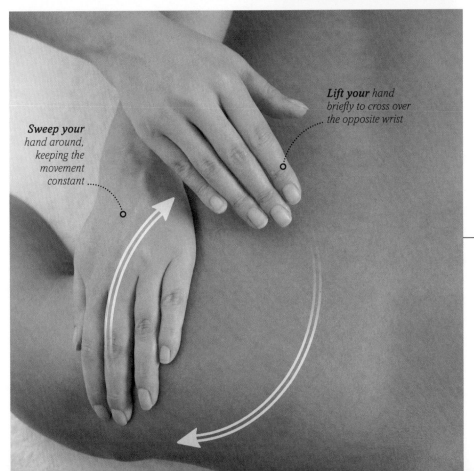

Sweep your hand around, keeping the movement constant

Lift your hand briefly to cross over the opposite wrist

— WITH WHOLE HAND

Circle over large areas such as the shoulders and back using your entire palm. Begin with your hands at opposite sides of the circle and move them clockwise, avoiding bony areas such as the spine.

(2)

Lift one hand to cross over the opposite wrist when it reaches it, keeping your other hand in contact with the body as you do so to ensure constant movement and contact. Do several repetitions on one shoulder before repeating the action on the opposite side.

CRISS-CROSS

WHEN TO USE
After oiling, or
deep strokes

GOOD FOR
Warming and
soothing

PRESSURE
Moderate to
deep

This linear push-and-pull action is a light, soothing effleurage stroke, though it can also be applied more deeply, as a kneading petrissage action. As the tissues are squeezed and stretched, blood flow to the area is boosted, making this a very relaxing and warming stroke that can be used as preparation for deeper strokes. It can also be done after vigorous deep tissue work to soothe the tissues. Criss-cross is typically done on larger areas, such as the back; thighs; and, more lightly, on the abdomen.

HAND CRISS-CROSS

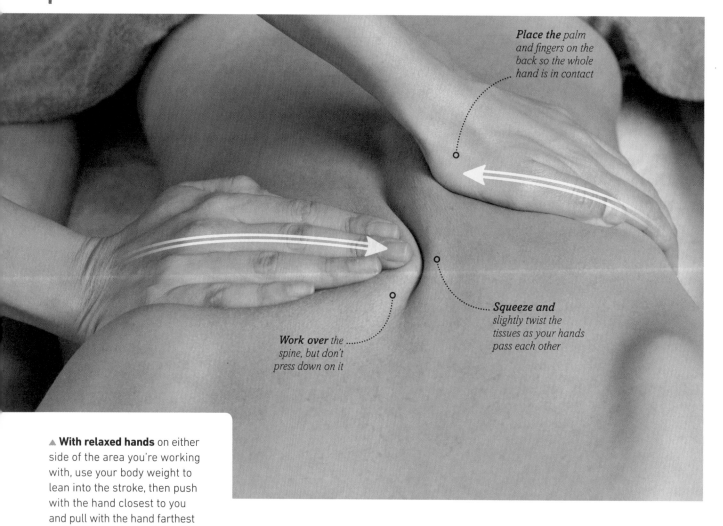

Place the palm and fingers on the back so the whole hand is in contact

Squeeze and slightly twist the tissues as your hands pass each other

Work over the spine, but don't press down on it

▲ **With relaxed hands** on either side of the area you're working with, use your body weight to lean into the stroke, then push with the hand closest to you and pull with the hand farthest from you, squeezing tissues at the center as your hands cross over. Repeat back and forth.

"Squeezing and compressing the tissues is extremely relaxing and warming."

FOREARM CRISS-CROSS

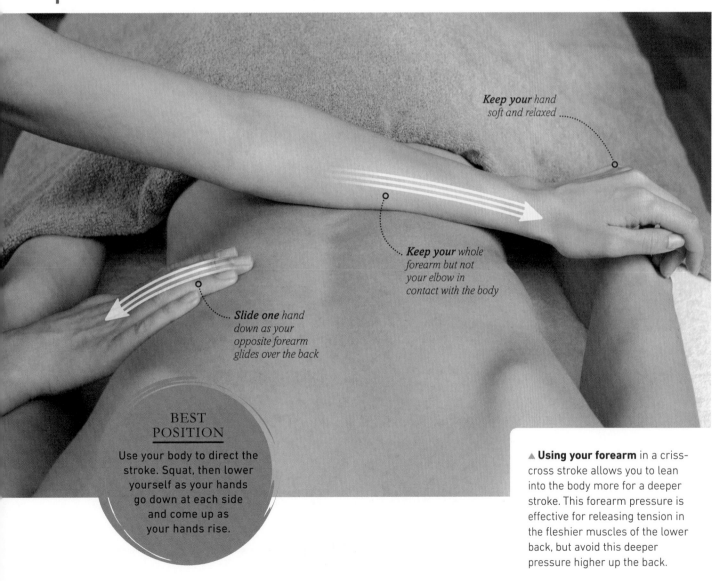

Keep your hand soft and relaxed

Keep your whole forearm but not your elbow in contact with the body

Slide one hand down as your opposite forearm glides over the back

BEST POSITION

Use your body to direct the stroke. Squat, then lower yourself as your hands go down at each side and come up as your hands rise.

▲ **Using your forearm** in a criss-cross stroke allows you to lean into the body more for a deeper stroke. This forearm pressure is effective for releasing tension in the fleshier muscles of the lower back, but avoid this deeper pressure higher up the back.

FIGURE-EIGHT

WHEN TO USE
After effleurage, predeep strokes

GOOD FOR
Stretching and warming tissues

PRESSURE
Moderate to deep (light on spine)

This technique moves and stretches the tissues in different directions. It is best done after initial warm-up strokes, and the stretching action is helpful preparation for deeper tissue work. It can be done with reinforced hands over fleshy areas, or your hands can work separately to incorporate a crosswise stretch of tissues over the whole length of the back, shoulder, and hip.

REINFORCED HANDS

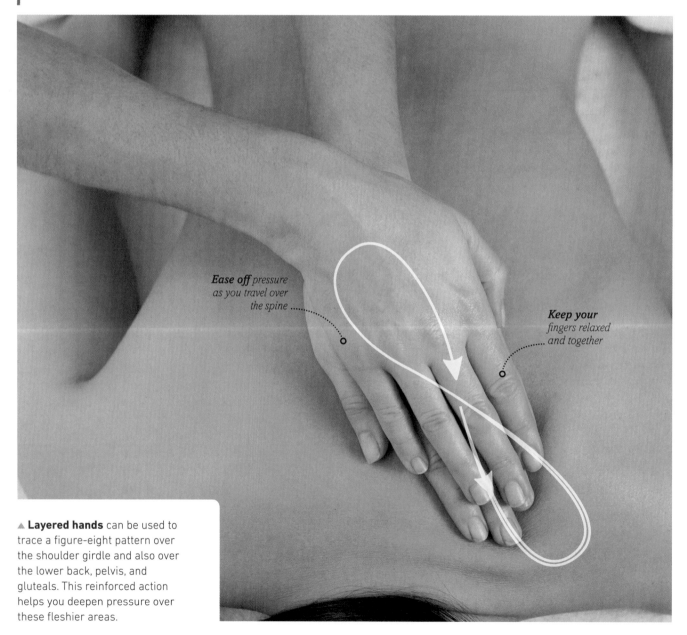

Ease off pressure as you travel over the spine

Keep your fingers relaxed and together

▲ **Layered hands** can be used to trace a figure-eight pattern over the shoulder girdle and also over the lower back, pelvis, and gluteals. This reinforced action helps you deepen pressure over these fleshier areas.

SINGLE HANDS

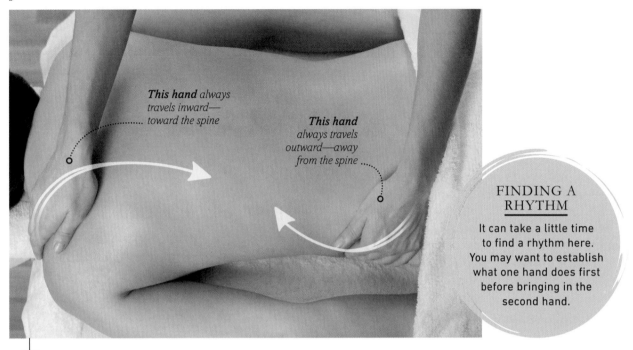

This hand always travels inward— toward the spine

This hand always travels outward—away from the spine

FINDING A RHYTHM

It can take a little time to find a rhythm here. You may want to establish what one hand does first before bringing in the second hand.

(1) **Squatting side-on**, place one hand on the far shoulder, the other at the base of the back on the far side. Move your hands together, pulling up tissues with the one near the shoulder, pushing them with your hand near the hip.

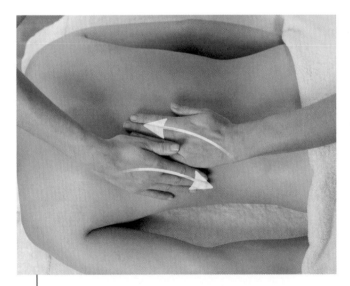

(2) **Glide both hands** toward each other, swinging them around so that the fingers face, until they meet in the midback. Lighten the pressure as you travel over the middle of the back.

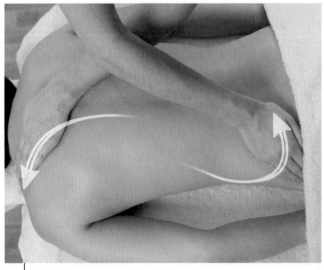

(3) **Cross your arms** and glide each hand to the opposite end of the back in a flowing figure-eight pattern. Swap sides to repeat on the opposite side of the back.

DEEP STROKES

WHEN TO USE
After warm-up techniques

GOOD FOR
Releasing chronic tension

PRESSURE
Deep

Working deeply into the tissues and fascia allows you to target areas that often carry tension, such as the back, trapezius, and leg muscles. Using different parts of your body or reinforced hands to apply the pressure helps protect your wrists and hands and allows you to lean in and use your body weight to intensify pressure. Warm and prepare the tissues first with lighter strokes and return to lighter strokes afterward to soothe the body. Deep strokes should always be done very slowly and sensitively.

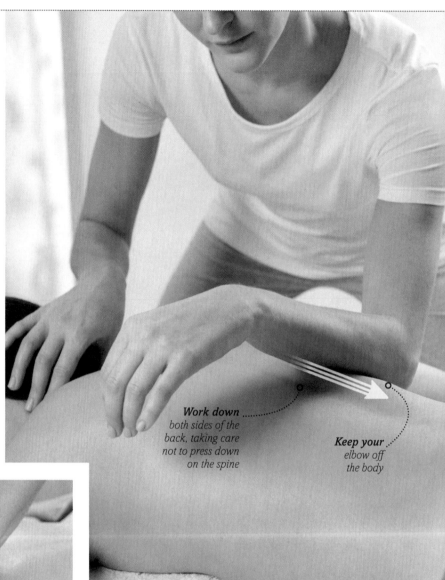

Work down both sides of the back, taking care not to press down on the spine

Keep your elbow off the body

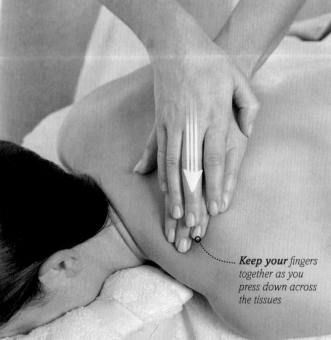

Keep your fingers together as you press down across the tissues

— REINFORCED HANDS

◀ **Place one hand** on top of the other to deepen pressure and also stabilize and protect your wrist and fingers. This is a good technique for working across tissues—for example, over the trapezius muscles of the shoulders.

NOTICE RESPONSES

Be attuned to the receiver's responses. Check that the receiver is happy with the pressure and ease up or go deeper as needed.

FOREARM PRESSURE

▲ **Pressing down with** your forearm helps you to apply deep pressure over large areas such as the back. Squat down and use your body weight to deepen the pressure, easing off over the kidney area in the midback and going deeper over the gluteals and trapezius muscles.

CUPPED HANDS ▬

This technique warms the calf ▶ muscle tissues and is a useful sports' warm-up, though avoid it with conditions such as DVT. Work up the calf, pressing in with the heel of the hands, releasing, then moving along and repeating. Stop before the knee and glide back down.

SIDE OF THE HAND

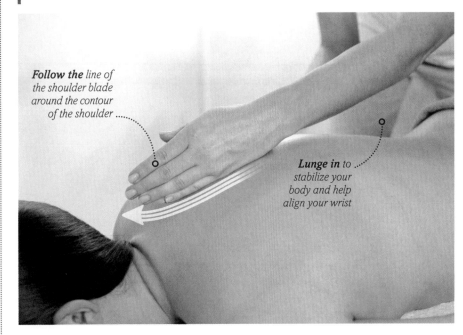

Follow the line of the shoulder blade around the contour of the shoulder ·····

Lunge in to ····· stabilize your body and help align your wrist

▲ **The side of your hand** can be used to access the small, tight area between the spine and scapula. Place your other hand on the shoulder for support and to comfort the receiver and connect them to their body and your touch.

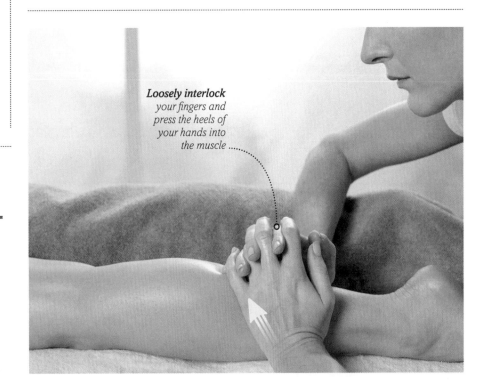

Loosely interlock your fingers and press the heels of your hands into the muscle ·····

FEATHERING

WHEN TO USE
To finish an area
or whole session

GOOD FOR
Relaxing and
de-energizing

PRESSURE
Extremely
light

This very light touch gently stimulates the nerves rather than acting on muscles, and can feel very relaxing. But it can also tickle, so it is best done on less sensitive areas such as the back, leg, forearm, and scalp, once the receiver is already relaxed. It signals the end of a massage to a particular area or the end of a complete session and draws energy down.

| FINGERTIP FEATHERING

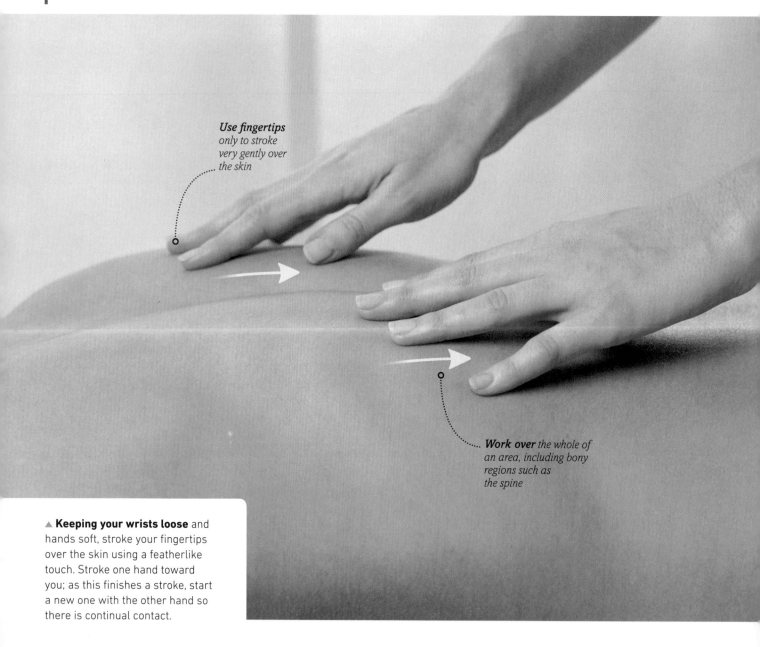

Use fingertips only to stroke very gently over the skin

Work over the whole of an area, including bony regions such as the spine

▲ **Keeping your wrists loose** and hands soft, stroke your fingertips over the skin using a featherlike touch. Stroke one hand toward you; as this finishes a stroke, start a new one with the other hand so there is continual contact.

| BACKS OF THE HANDS

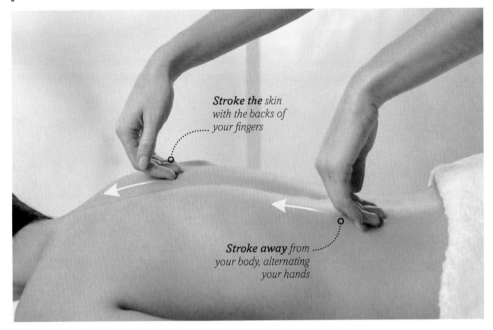

Stroke the skin
with the backs of
your fingers

Stroke away from
your body, alternating
your hands

▲ **Feathering with the backs** of your hands creates
a slightly tingly sensation that can be used for a more
sensual effect—for example, if massaging a partner.

READING REACTIONS

Be sensitive to how
the receiver is feeling. For
some, feathering simply
irritates and tickles rather
than soothes and is
best avoided.

◀ **ALTERNATIVE METHOD**
Feather over a towel to
keep the receiver warm
at the end of a session.

BASIC TECHNIQUES
PETRISSAGE

Petrissage techniques are compression strokes to the fleshy, muscular areas of the body that are done after the tissues have been warmed up with lighter effleurage strokes. Petrissage works along and across muscle fibers, engaging the deeper layer of muscles. The action of squeezing and twisting and then releasing works deeply into an area to release stickiness in the fascia; boosts circulation; and encourages the natural elimination of waste products from the tissues via the lymphatic system. The techniques should be carried out in a steady, continuous rhythm. Some effleurage movements, where tissues are worked into more deeply or squeezed against each other, can cross over into petrissage techniques.

WRINGING

WHEN TO USE
After warming effleurage

GOOD FOR
Boosting circulation

PRESSURE
Moderate

This is a compression "push–pull" movement incorporating a twist that should be done on lightly oiled skin to avoid an unpleasant stretch. The smooth, rhythmic action is done on fleshy areas such as the torso and thighs. If you feel a knot of tension, home in with some finger and thumb kneading (see p.60). Wringing can also be done with the forearms, working side-on as shown here, turning your body rhythmically first toward the head and then toward the lower limbs to twist the flesh.

DEEP RELEASE

This energetic action can feel very releasing. Ask the receiver how they feel and go deeper if they are enjoying the pressure.

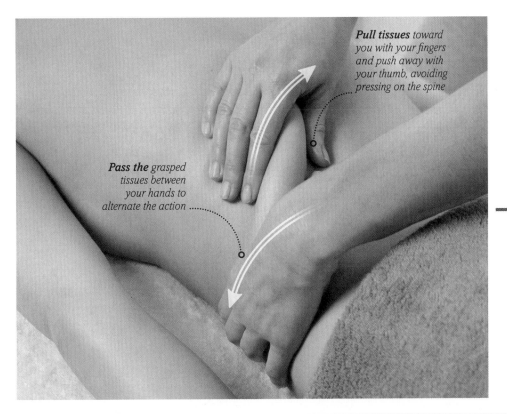

Pull tissues toward you with your fingers and push away with your thumb, avoiding pressing on the spine

Pass the grasped tissues between your hands to alternate the action

WITH THUMBS SPLAYED

◂ **Wringing the tissues** with fingers and splayed thumbs creates a vigorous twisting and squeezing action. Move up and down an area, working on the opposite (contralateral) side of the back. Overusing this technique can strain your thumbs, so use it with caution.

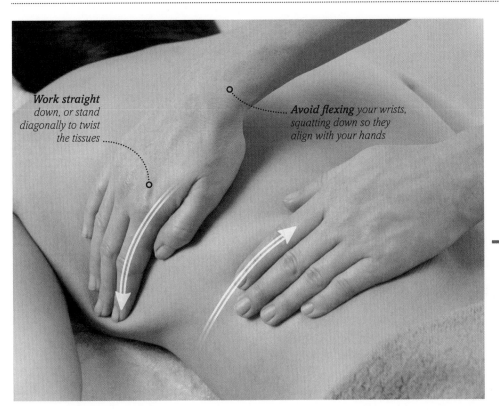

Work straight down, or stand diagonally to twist the tissues

Avoid flexing your wrists, squatting down so they align with your hands

WITH THUMBS TUCKED IN

◂ **Keeping your thumbs** next to your fingers achieves a gentler twist but protects your thumbs from strain. Sway from side to side to control the movement from your body rather than from your wrists and hands.

KNUCKLING

WHEN TO USE
Usually near the
end of a session

GOOD FOR
Relaxing and
revitalizing

PRESSURE
Light
to deep

This technique involves holding your hands in soft, relaxed fists, your fingers curled at the second joint as if holding something loosely, then massaging with your knuckles (using just a small amount of oil) to stimulate blood flow to an area. The action can be slow, rhythmic, and relaxing—as is the case with circular knuckling done on sensitive regions—or more energizing, stretching tissues as you work over fleshy areas.

CIRCULAR

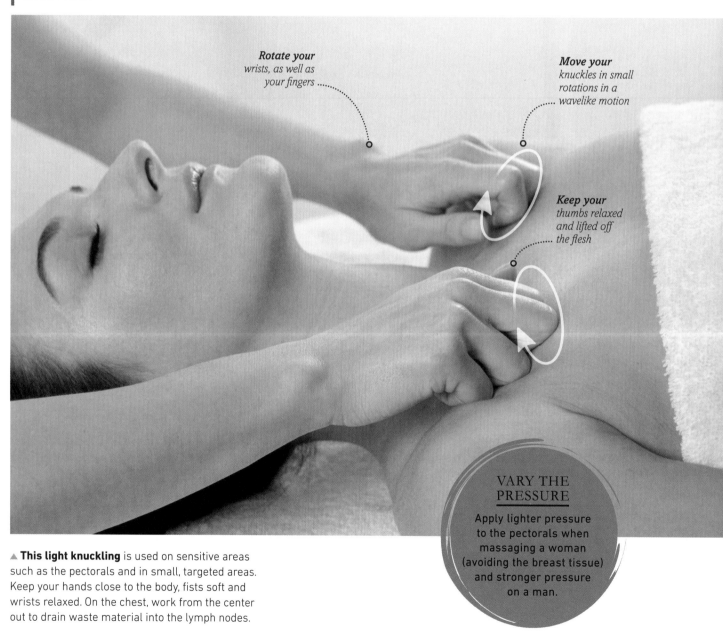

Rotate your wrists, as well as your fingers

Move your knuckles in small rotations in a wavelike motion

Keep your thumbs relaxed and lifted off the flesh

VARY THE PRESSURE

Apply lighter pressure to the pectorals when massaging a woman (avoiding the breast tissue) and stronger pressure on a man.

▲ **This light knuckling** is used on sensitive areas such as the pectorals and in small, targeted areas. Keep your hands close to the body, fists soft and wrists relaxed. On the chest, work from the center out to drain waste material into the lymph nodes.

| LINEAR

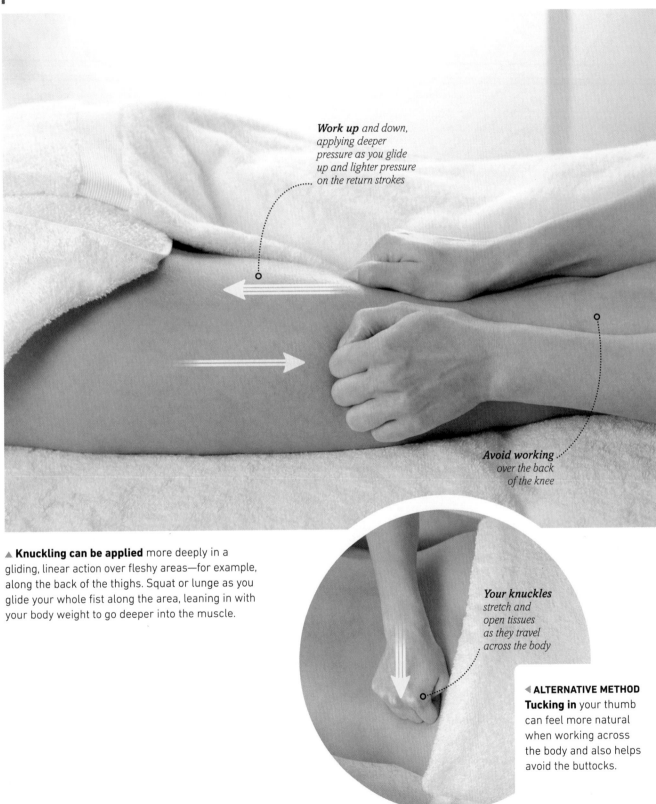

Work up and down, applying deeper pressure as you glide up and lighter pressure on the return strokes

Avoid working over the back of the knee

Your knuckles stretch and open tissues as they travel across the body

▲ **Knuckling can be applied** more deeply in a gliding, linear action over fleshy areas—for example, along the back of the thighs. Squat or lunge as you glide your whole fist along the area, leaning in with your body weight to go deeper into the muscle.

◀ **ALTERNATIVE METHOD Tucking in** your thumb can feel more natural when working across the body and also helps avoid the buttocks.

KNEADING

WHEN TO USE
After initial
warm-up strokes

GOOD FOR
Tension release
in tissues

PRESSURE
Moderate
to deep

This petrissage technique using fingers, thumbs, and sometimes the heel of the hand pulls, lifts, and pushes tissues in a kneading action, working into the muscles to release stickiness in the fascia and relieve tension and pain. Kneading can be a useful technique for working into smaller areas—for example, the fleshy area at the top of the trapezius or between the scapula and spine.

TWO-HANDED KNEADING

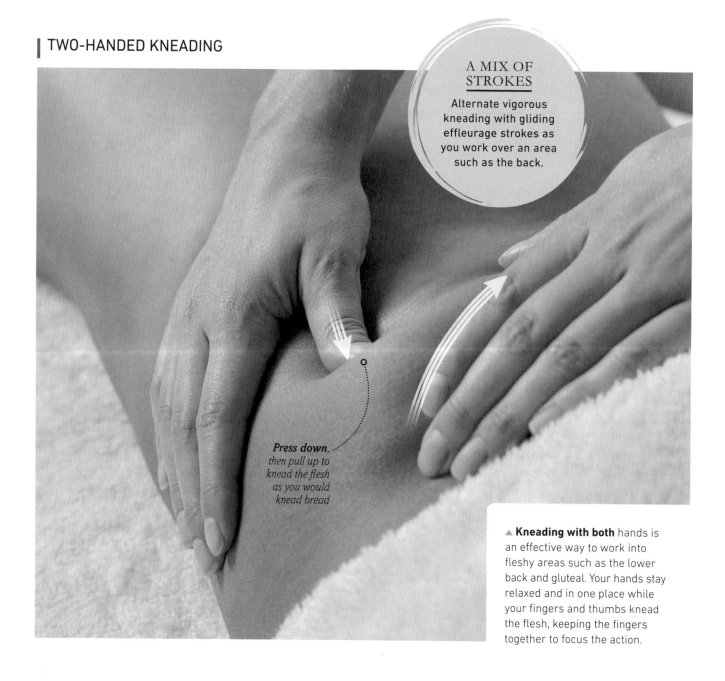

A MIX OF STROKES

Alternate vigorous kneading with gliding effleurage strokes as you work over an area such as the back.

Press down,
then pull up to
knead the flesh
as you would
knead bread

▲ **Kneading with both** hands is an effective way to work into fleshy areas such as the lower back and gluteal. Your hands stay relaxed and in one place while your fingers and thumbs knead the flesh, keeping the fingers together to focus the action.

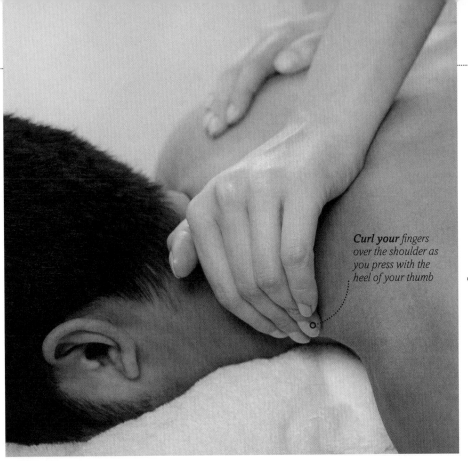

Curl your fingers over the shoulder as you press with the heel of your thumb

USING THE HEEL

◀ **The heel of your thumb** can be used to knead into the curve of the shoulder, allowing you to knead deeply into the shoulder area without putting pressure on your thumbs. Press into the flesh with the heel of your thumb, not the whole palm, avoiding pressing on the spine.

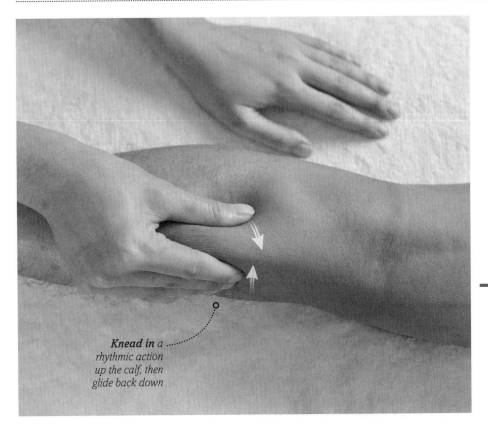

Knead in a rhythmic action up the calf, then glide back down

ONE-HANDED KNEADING

◀ **For smaller**, fleshy parts of the body—such as the calf, arm, or shoulder—knead with one hand only. Lift the flesh with your thumb and fingers, then use your thumb to roll it across toward your fingers.

SKIN ROLLING

WHEN TO USE
After warming strokes

GOOD FOR
Releasing tension

PRESSURE
Light to moderate

This technique lifts and rolls tissues to help release adhesions between the skin and fascia. Skin rolling is useful for targeting areas of tightness that can cause pain—for example, between the spine and shoulder blades or in the erector spinae (the muscles along the back). Let the fingers sink in to work tissues slowly and release tension gradually.

NO-OIL TECHNIQUE

It is best to do skin rolling on dry skin, without oil, so that the fingers can lift and stretch the tissues without slipping.

Gently squeeze, lift, and roll the tissues toward you, being careful not to pinch

Keep your *fingers together, without tension, as you grasp a small mound of tissue between fingers and thumbs*

OVER FLESHY AREAS

▲ **With relaxed hands** and wrists, move and stretch tissues gently in a push–pull rolling action with fingers and thumbs. Release and repeat on the next section of skin, moving slowly across an area. If working up from the sacrum, travel up each side in turn, standing on the side you are working on.

◀ **ALTERNATIVE VIEW**
Sink your thumbs in as your fingers roll the flesh toward you.

"Sense areas of tension and work into these parts of the body."

OVER BONY AREAS

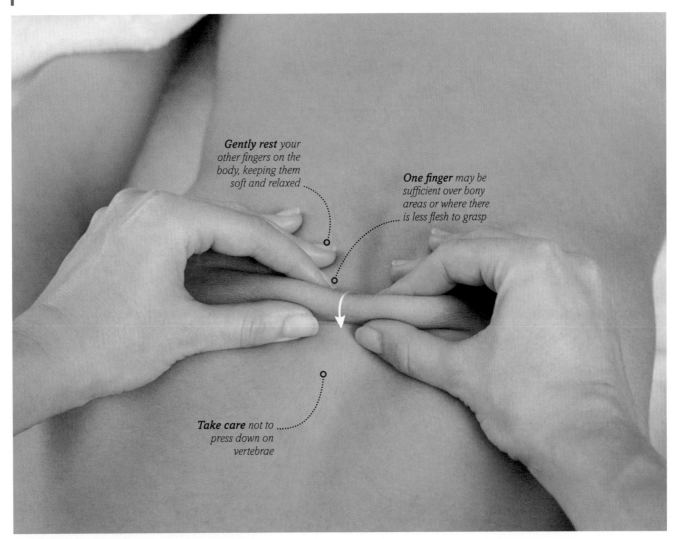

Gently rest your other fingers on the body, keeping them soft and relaxed

One finger may be sufficient over bony areas or where there is less flesh to grasp

Take care not to press down on vertebrae

▲ **Skin rolling can be done** over bony areas such as the spine as you lift and pull rather than push down. To work down the back, lean over from the head as far as is comfortable, then move to the side as you work down to the base of the back.

BASIC TECHNIQUES
PERCUSSION

Also known as tapotement, percussion techniques are "wake-up, break-up" strokes. These dynamic, vigorous strokes with a steady staccato rhythm are used either to wake up the body—for example, at the end of a massage to bring the receiver out of a deeply relaxed state, or in preparation for a sporting event—or to break up areas of congestion. Percussion is usually avoided over bony areas and the neck and should not be done over injuries, broken veins, damaged skin, or on the abdomen.

RHYTHMIC STRIKES

WHEN TO USE	GOOD FOR	PRESSURE
Near the end of a massage session	**Energizing**	**Light to moderate**

These percussive strokes boost blood flow to an area, helping to reawaken and energize the body. Percussion is not usually done over bony areas, though the cupping technique on page 66 can be helpful over the midback to loosen catarrh. Keep the wrists soft and springy as you tap, drum, or lightly strike.

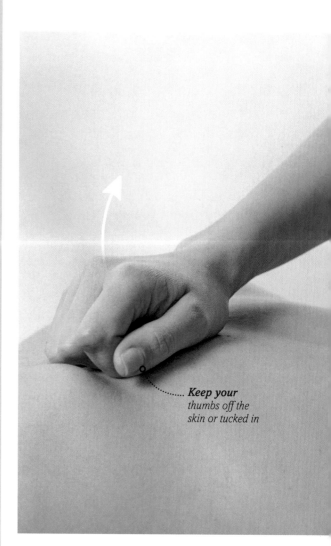

Keep your *thumbs off the skin or tucked in*

"Rhythmic strikes boost blood flow to the tissues and energize the body."

HACKING

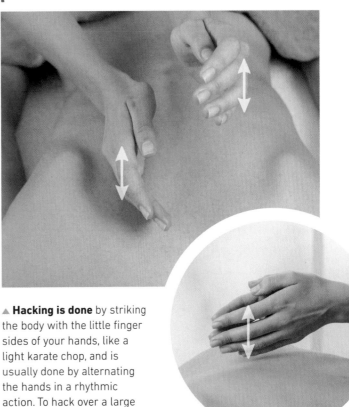

▲ **Hacking is done** by striking the body with the little finger sides of your hands, like a light karate chop, and is usually done by alternating the hands in a rhythmic action. To hack over a large area such as the back, stand in a squat and lunge your body from side to side to direct the action.

▲ **ALTERNATIVE METHOD** You can also hack with your hands joined. Hold them loosely rather than tightly pressed to keep them relaxed, fingertips gently touching.

PUMMELING

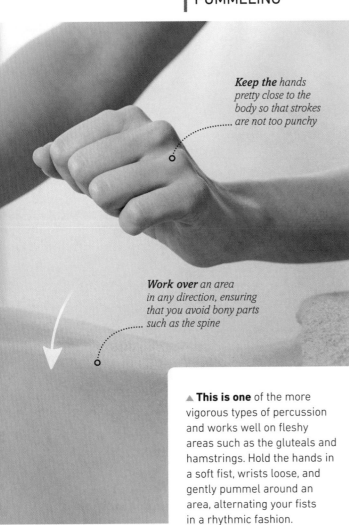

Keep the *hands pretty close to the body so that strokes are not too punchy*

Work over *an area in any direction, ensuring that you avoid bony parts such as the spine*

▲ **This is one** of the more vigorous types of percussion and works well on fleshy areas such as the gluteals and hamstrings. Hold the hands in a soft fist, wrists loose, and gently pummel around an area, alternating your fists in a rhythmic fashion.

CONTINUED ▶

RHYTHMIC STRIKES *continued*

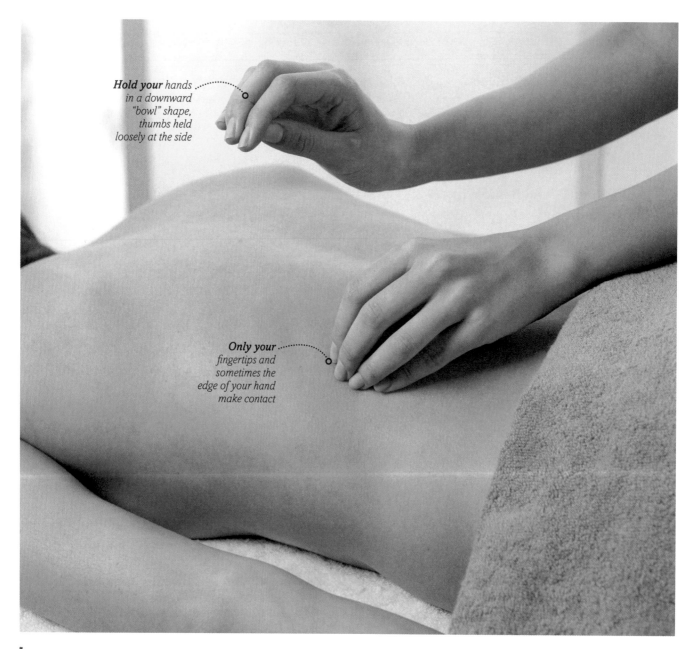

Hold your hands in a downward "bowl" shape, thumbs held loosely at the side

Only your fingertips and sometimes the edge of your hand make contact

CUPPING

▲ **Loosely cupping** your hands to pummel feels lighter than other types of percussion. This rhythmic stroke is often used over the ribcage area of the back to help loosen congestion. It can also be done with the receiver seated and clothed, leaning over a chair.

TAPPING —

Drumming your fingers ▷
lightly, like raindrops, feels
energizing and stimulating
but is also relaxing, so it is
slightly more calming than
other percussions. This
lighter stroke is often done
on the scalp and over the
shoulders (avoiding the
neck) as part of a head
massage, or, more gently
still, around the eye sockets
to clear sinus congestion.

Keep your
palms
still as you
tap your
fingertips
in a gentle
pitter-patter
action

Alternate your
hands in a
rhythmic pattern ....

◀ **ALTERNATIVE METHOD**
Tap all the fingers of your
hand together for a slower,
very relaxing sensation.

FINAL STROKES

Percussion signals
the closing stages of
a massage. It may be
followed with feathering
and the calm placing
of hands in a
final hold.

BASIC TECHNIQUES
VIBRATIONS

Vibrations can involve a fairly vigorous shaking of a limb or a rocking movement of the body to loosen restrictions at joints, or they can be smaller "shaking" actions, usually done with the fingertips, to target specific areas of tension that may be discovered when working on a particular part of the body. With the more subtle fingertip shaking, the aim is to vibrate the layers beneath the skin, rather than the skin itself, to help break up sticky adhesions in the tissues.

SHAKING

WHEN TO USE
Before massaging a limb

GOOD FOR
Helping receiver to let go

MOVEMENT
Gentle to fairly vigorous

This assisted movement helps loosen a limb (usually an arm or hand) and release tension, making it easier to work with the relaxed tissues. Shaking is helpful before working on a limb, or between strokes if you sense tension. Avoid using oil, or use minimal oil, to stop you sliding and rubbing across the skin.

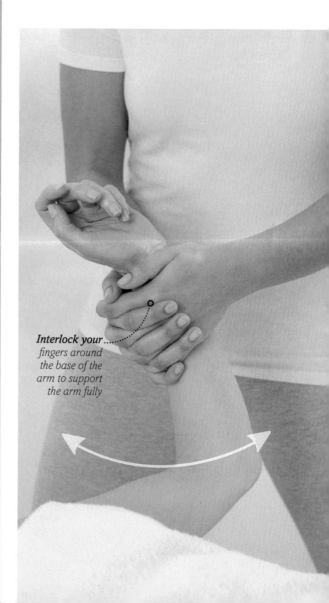

Interlock your fingers around the base of the arm to support the arm fully

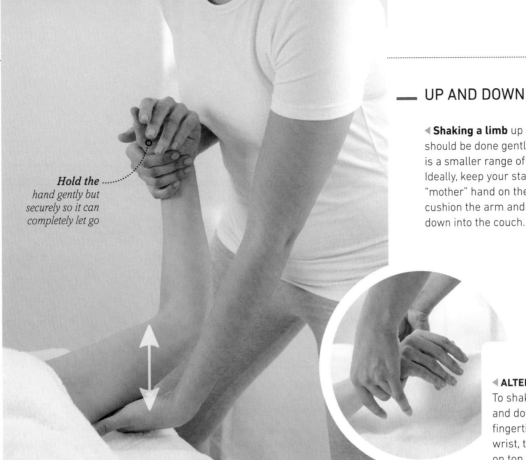

Hold the
*hand gently but
securely so it can
completely let go*

__ UP AND DOWN

◀ **Shaking a limb** up and down should be done gently, as there is a smaller range of motion here. Ideally, keep your stabilizing "mother" hand on the couch to cushion the arm and stop it hitting down into the couch.

◀ **ALTERNATIVE METHOD**
To shake a hand up and down, put your fingertips under the wrist, thumbs lightly on top, and shake.

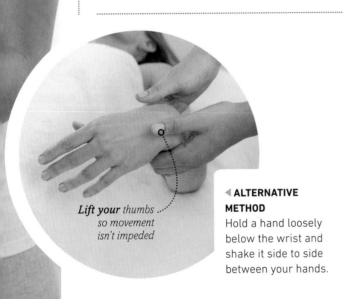

*Lift your thumbs
so movement
isn't impeded*

◀ **ALTERNATIVE METHOD**
Hold a hand loosely below the wrist and shake it side to side between your hands.

__ SIDE TO SIDE

◀ **Shaking a limb** or hand from side to side can be done gently or pretty vigorously. Sense the range of motion and go gently if there is more stiffness. Shake for a few moments, until you feel the limb or hand relax.

▌FINGERTIP SHAKING

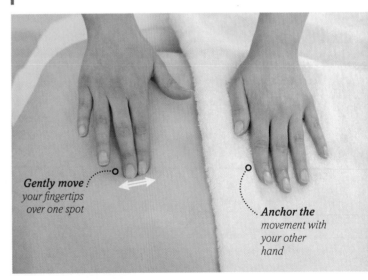

*Gently move
your fingertips
over one spot*

*Anchor the
movement with
your other
hand*

▲ **This small vibrating** movement is carried out by sinking your fingers into the flesh to vibrate the tissues under the skin. Work across the muscle fibers, sensing in which direction they are most responsive to moving.

ROCKING

WHEN TO USE
Start of session

GOOD FOR
Connecting with
the receiver

MOVEMENT
Light

Rocking, or pulsing, is a rhythmic movement done at the start of a session over towels to help you connect with the receiver and introduce touch. It can also relax areas of tension or loosen joints— for example, in the shoulders or legs—without straining yourself. Done slowly, it is very relaxing; more quickly, it is energizing and invigorating.

ROCKING WITH ONE HAND —

Keeping one hand in a ▶ stationary position on the sacrum to anchor the body, place your other hand next to it and gently push the body away with your top hand, allowing the body to roll back to you in a small, gentle rocking action. Work up, then down the torso with your top hand in this way. Swap hands and use your lower hand to rock down, then back up the legs.

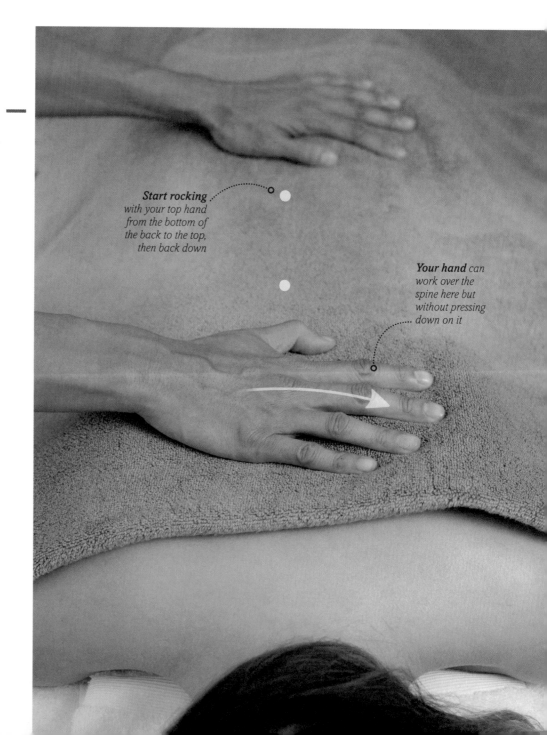

Start rocking with your top hand from the bottom of the back to the top, then back down

Your hand can work over the spine here but without pressing down on it

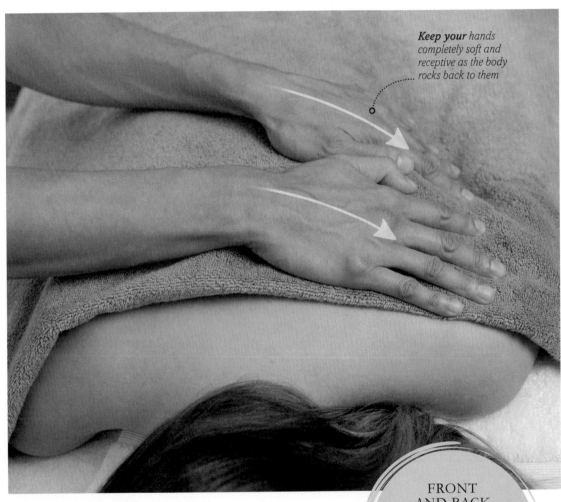

Keep your hands *completely soft and receptive as the body rocks back to them*

ROCKING WITH TWO HANDS

▲ **Rock with both hands** to release tension in the shoulder. Place your hands either on the far side of the torso or on the side closest to you (which can put less strain on you), avoiding the spine. Push the body away, allowing it to rock back. Do this several times, building a steady rhythm.

FRONT AND BACK

You can rock the torso with the receiver lying either face down (prone) or turned onto their back facing up (supine).

BASIC TECHNIQUES
PRESSURE

These pressure moves can be useful for sensing and working on areas of tension and tenderness and trigger points (see pp.130–133). Before using the techniques, make sure you have softened the tissues first with slow, releasing strokes; otherwise, the pressure could be painful and cause the body to tense rather than release. You also need to take care of your thumbs and fingers when applying pressure in this way. Try using the side of your thumb or the relaxed pads of your fingers (not the tips), and where possible apply pressure by resting your other arm, hand, or finger over the working hand or finger as you lean in.

STATIC AND CIRCULAR PRESSURE

WHEN TO USE	GOOD FOR	PRESSURE
After effleurage or deep petrissage	Identifying areas of tension	Moderate to deep

These small, slow movements are done mainly with your thumb but can also be applied with your forearm or, with great care, your elbow. When applying static pressure, slowly increase the depth so you can feel a gradual softening and release of the tissues, easing back on the pressure if you sense the tissues are beginning to tense. Circular pressures work over a slightly larger area, making small, circular movements to the tissues beneath the skin.

STATIC THUMB PRESSURE

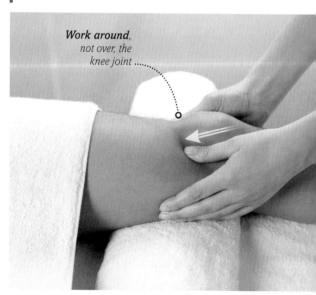

Work around, not over, the knee joint

▲ **Using your thumbs** independently allows you to apply pressure more gently around sensitive areas such as the knees and elbow joints. Apply pressure in the fleshier area around the joint.

STATIC ELBOW PRESSURE

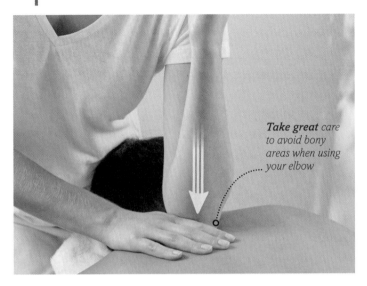

*Take **great** care to avoid bony areas when using your elbow*

▲ **Use sharper elbow** pressure mainly on men and over very developed muscles only, for example, to release the gluteals or trapezius. The elbow is less sensitive, so you are unlikely to sense tensing up.

STATIC FOREARM PRESSURE

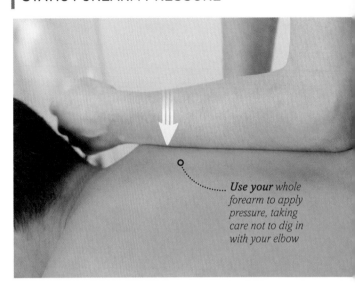

*Use **your** whole forearm to apply pressure, taking care not to dig in with your elbow*

▲ **Applying pressure** with your forearm lets you use your body weight to work into the tissues without straining your body. You may need to lower the bed to facilitate this deeper tissue work.

STATIC PRESSURE WITH REINFORCED THUMBS

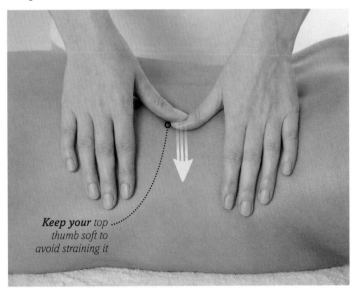

*Keep **your** top thumb soft to avoid straining it*

▲ **With your "sensing" thumb** soft and relaxed on the body (avoiding the spine), place your other thumb on top to apply pressure. This reinforced action protects your bottom thumb as you press down.

CIRCULAR PRESSURE WITH REINFORCED THUMBS

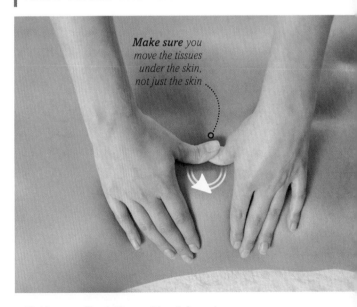

*Make **sure** you move the tissues under the skin, not just the skin*

▲ **Making small rotations** with reinforced thumbs helps release tension over a targeted area. Do this after some preliminary static pressure.

BASIC TECHNIQUES
PASSIVE MOVEMENTS

These gentle, slow stretches, rotations, flexions, and extensions allow you to explore and assess the receiver's natural range of motions before you work into an area. When you carry out these actions with the proper attention and respect, you will be able to feel where the receiver is holding tightness, signaling that you should ease off before gently repeating the move and feeling for a new point of resistance as tension is released. This gradual action helps the receiver to turn off their automatic protective responses and shows them what they can actually do. The receiver should not feel any pain—only release.

STRETCHES AND MOVES

WHEN TO USE	GOOD FOR	PRESSURE
At start or end of work to an area	Release of tension	Very gentle

Gentle stretches and assisted moves help the receiver let go before deeper tissue work, or can be done at the end of treating an area to see how far the tissues have released. Your actions should be smooth, slow, and without force. Work sensitively on the neck, or not at all if there has been an injury; avoid stretching hypermobile joints; and take care in pregnancy, when hormones soften cartilage, increasing the risk of injury.

FIGURE-EIGHT NECK MOVE

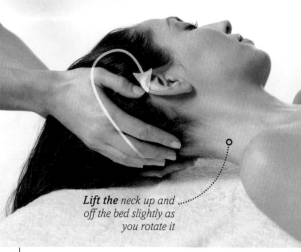

Lift the neck up and off the bed slightly as you rotate it

1 **Supporting the head** securely in your hands, start to move the neck very gently over to one side, feeling for the point of resistance.

ARM STRETCH

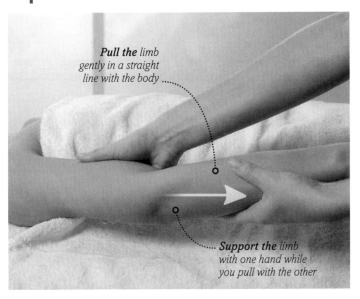

Pull the limb gently in a straight line with the body

Support the limb with one hand while you pull with the other

▲ **Ask the receiver** to relax completely, then use your body weight to pull the limb back gently until you feel some resistance.

NECK STRETCH

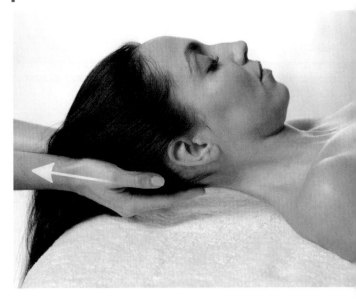

▲ **Place your fingers** under the bony occipital ridge to cradle the head, then lean back, applying a little traction until you feel the neck gently stretch.

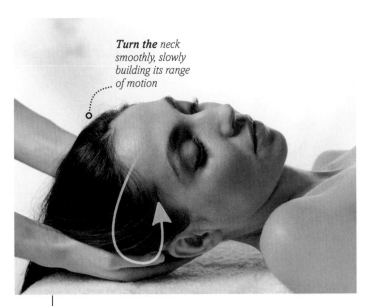

Turn the neck smoothly, slowly building its range of motion

② **Gently take** the neck over to the opposite side in a subtle figure-eight movement. Repeat this action a few times, ensuring that movements are small, slow, and predictable.

PASSING A LIMB

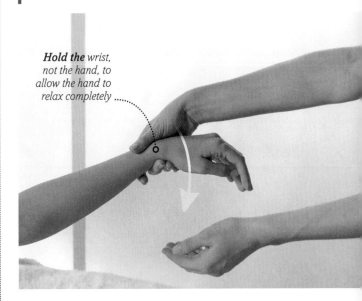

Hold the wrist, not the hand, to allow the hand to relax completely

▲ **Pass the stretched limb** back and forth from one hand to the other in a slow, fluid movement to help the receiver completely let go.

ROTATIONS

WHEN TO USE
Before working
on a limb or area

GOOD FOR
Encouraging
relaxation

MOVEMENT
Circular

Rotations are passive movements that are done extremely slowly to take, for example, a tight leg, arm, neck, or shoulder through its range of motion before you work more deeply into the area. The slow, supportive action helps you asséss the range of motion and also encourages the receiver to relax and release held-in tension. It's important that you feel completely relaxed yourself and focused while carrying out rotations.

| HEAD ROTATION

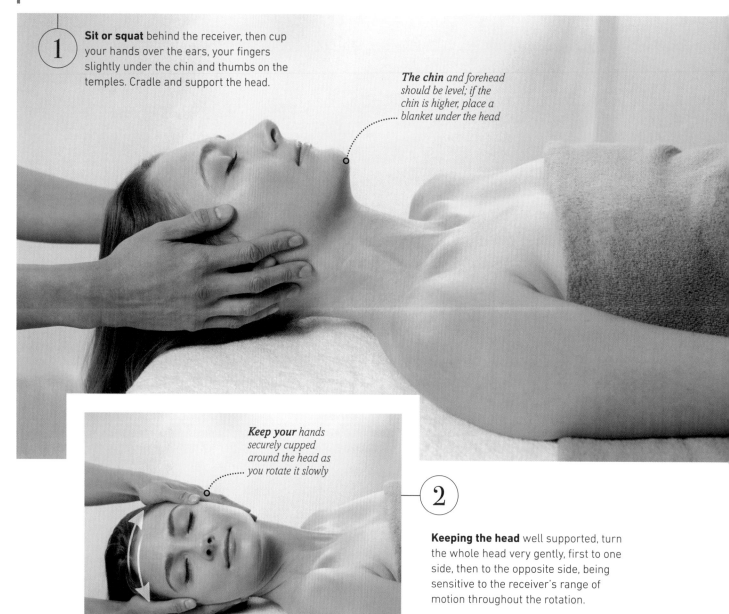

1 **Sit or squat** behind the receiver, then cup your hands over the ears, your fingers slightly under the chin and thumbs on the temples. Cradle and support the head.

The chin and forehead should be level; if the chin is higher, place a blanket under the head

Keep your hands securely cupped around the head as you rotate it slowly

2 **Keeping the head** well supported, turn the whole head very gently, first to one side, then to the opposite side, being sensitive to the receiver's range of motion throughout the rotation.

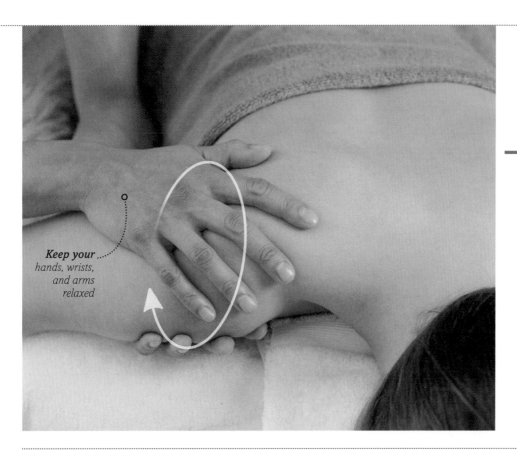

Keep your hands, wrists, and arms relaxed

SHOULDER ROTATION

◀ **This rotation** is done specifically on the shoulder. With one hand supporting the shoulder from below and the top hand covering the top of the shoulder, gently lift and rotate, working rhythmically and slowly in both directions.

HAND AND FINGER ROTATION

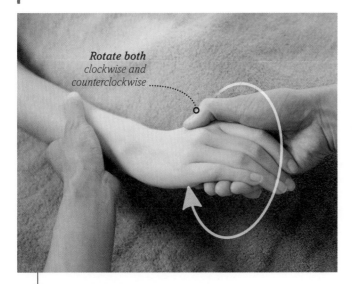

Rotate both clockwise and counterclockwise

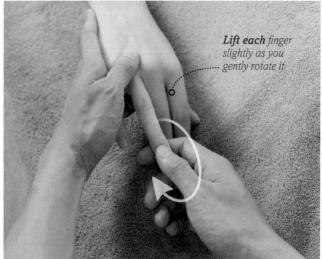

Lift each finger slightly as you gently rotate it

1 **Keeping the arm low**, support the forearm, holding it loosely to avoid transferring tension, while holding the hand in your other hand. Rotate the wrist joint gently in a small circular motion.

2 **After several wrist rotations**, move to the fingers, rotating each one in turn. Hold the hand at the joints and rotate each finger at its tip, keeping your own wrist straight to avoid any strain.

WHOLE-BODY MASSAGE

A holistic whole-body massage amalgamates the basic Swedish techniques (pp.38–77) into one flowing, seamless massage. The following sequence can form the starting point of a practice, allowing adaptations to be built in to address areas of concern. Here, gliding, oil-spreading effleurage strokes travel over the body, while kneading petrissage softens tissues before applying deeper targeted strokes. Starting with the back, each area of the body is worked on methodically, moving slowly at an even pace and maintaining constant contact. Pressure builds and subsides to stimulate and relax, and minimum disruption allows the receiver to relax deeply and immerse themselves fully in the massage.

KEY

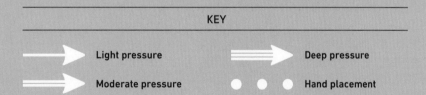

→ **Light pressure**   ⇒ **Deep pressure**

→ **Moderate pressure**   ● ● ● **Hand placement**

PUTTING IT ALL TOGETHER

When you feel ready to put your knowledge of the basic techniques into practice in a whole-body massage, take some time first to consider how the techniques will come together and the practical elements of the massage. Knowing which techniques to use to keep the massage flowing and how to position a person, place towels, and help them to change position with minimum disruption will all help make the massage enjoyable and relaxing for both you and the receiver.

WHAT TO THINK ABOUT

Before embarking on the step-by-step sequence on pages 82–107, run through this practical guide to ensure you feel prepped, confident, and relaxed.

A FLOWING MASSAGE

A full-body massage should feel effortlessly flowing for the receiver, your constant, reassuring touch allowing him or her to relax completely. How you link the strokes and build pressure so that each area you massage flows seamlessly into the next is key. Effleurage strokes are the foundation of a massage. These gliding strokes allow you to build depth and soften tissues gradually; they are returned to after deeper work to soothe tissues; and they are a useful tool for moving from one area to another. When moving around the table, maintaining contact at all times with the simple placement of a hand helps reassure the receiver and maintain flow. Keep an eye on the towels in case these are disturbed, adjusting them to ensure the modesty of the receiver throughout.

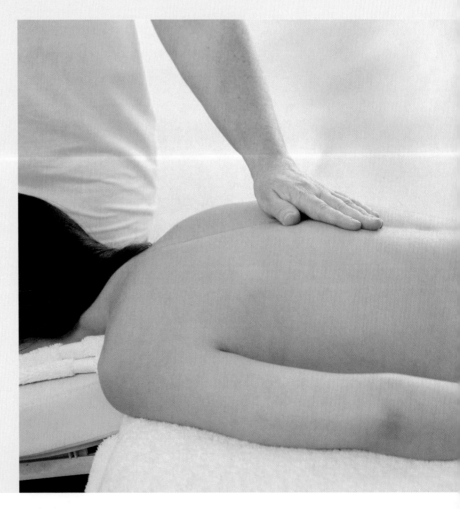

TIMING YOUR MASSAGE

A full-body massage is usually 1 hour long, though it can be up to 1 hour, 30 minutes. The easiest way to time it is to divide the body into sections and allocate an approximate amount of time for each area. This gives a rough guide, bearing in mind that you may need to adapt timings to meet particular requirements. For example, if someone has a lot of stiffness in the shoulders, you may want to spend more time on this area. This suggested timetable for a 1-hour massage offers a guide to be adapted as needed:

With the receiver prone (face down)
- Back, shoulders, and neck **20 minutes**
- Legs and feet **5 minutes** each

With the receiver supine (face up)
- Feet and legs **5 minutes** each
- Abdomen **5 minutes**
- Arms and hands **5 minutes** each
- Upper chest, neck, face, and head **5 minutes**

GETTING ONTO THE COUCH

Tell the receiver which items of clothing to take off and which to leave on: underwear is left on and other clothing (and jewelry and glasses) usually removed. Let them change in privacy, with a towel to wrap around them.

If the receiver can lie face down without help, ask them to pull the towel lengthwise over the top of the body like a blanket. Once he or she is in place, smooth the towel so it covers the shoulders. Place a second towel vertically, tucked under the first, to cover the legs and feet, then smooth this out. Place a folded towel or bolster under the ankles if there

◀ **CONSTANT CONTACT**
Keeping contact with the receiver throughout the massage ensures flow.

is space and tuck the lower towel into the underwear. Clean the feet with wipes or a washcloth, wiping your hands afterward. Make sure your hands are warm before you start.

TURNING OVER

When turning someone prone to supine, remove ankle support and ask the receiver to turn slowly toward you. Anchor the near side of the towel and lift the far side. Once turned, put support under the knees and head if needed.

CLOSING THE MASSAGE

Cover the receiver completely and leave them for a couple minutes, telling them to get up carefully before dressing. Once dressed, offer some water. Suggest they avoid washing for a while to reap the oils' benefits; advise them to drink lots of water and avoid heavy meals and alcohol that day to help detoxify; and, if you used one, give them their bespoke oil blend.

WHEN HELP IS NEEDED

If the receiver needs help getting off the couch at the end of the treatment, follow the steps below.

- If the receiver is lying face down, turn them so they are supine, or face up (see Turning over, above).
- Ask the receiver to put their arms over the top towel, then remove the towel over the legs and feet. Holding the towel on the near side of the couch, ask the receiver to roll toward you to lie on their side.
- Making sure the towel behind the back is secure, ask the receiver to swing their legs off the couch and to use their arms to push up into a sitting position, wrapping the towel around them.
- Allow the receiver to sit for at least a minute—offer some water now—before getting up.
- Securing the towel, help the receiver to get off the couch, maintaining their modesty at all times.

BACK, SHOULDERS, AND NECK

The back, shoulders, and neck are the largest area to be massaged and also hold a lot of tension, so a whole-body massage usually begins here and the most time is spent on this area. The focus is on the lower and upper back and shoulders rather than the midback, where you need to go gently over the kidneys. Start slowly to allow the receiver to calm their breathing and acclimatize to your touch.

BASIC TECHNIQUES USED
○ **Fan stroke, p.40**
○ **Figure-eight, p.50**

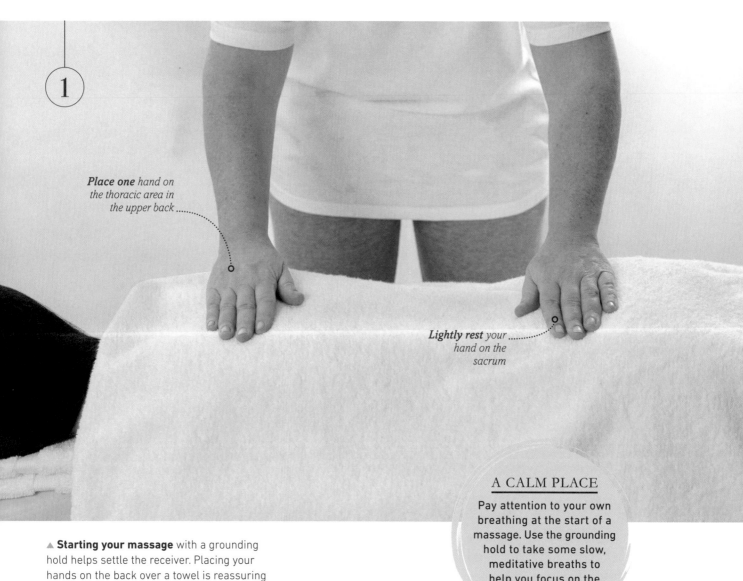

①

Place one hand on the thoracic area in the upper back

Lightly rest your hand on the sacrum

▲ **Starting your massage** with a grounding hold helps settle the receiver. Placing your hands on the back over a towel is reassuring and introduces your touch. As you hold this position, observe the receiver's breathing, waiting a few moments for the breath to calm.

A CALM PLACE

Pay attention to your own breathing at the start of a massage. Use the grounding hold to take some slow, meditative breaths to help you focus on the massage ahead.

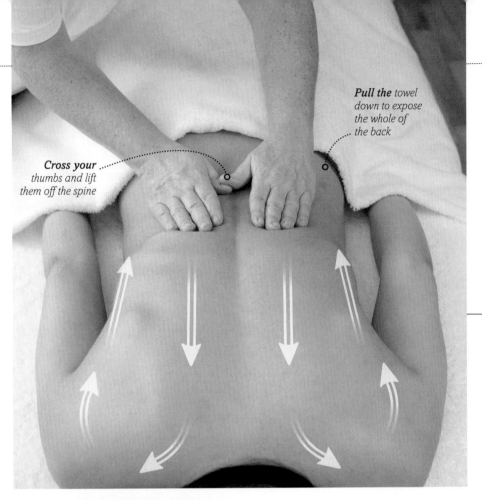

Cross your thumbs and lift them off the spine

Pull the towel down to expose the whole of the back

2

Start your work on the back with effleurage strokes to warm the tissues and release fascia from the muscles. Oil your hands (see p.32), then begin with one large fan stroke, spreading oil over the back. Glide your hands up, cup the shoulders, then sweep back down the sides of the body in a fan shape.

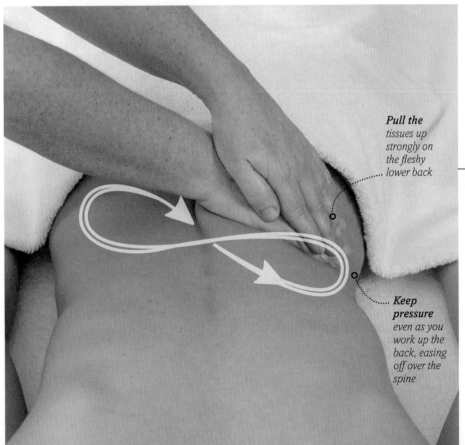

Pull the tissues up strongly on the fleshy lower back

Keep pressure even as you work up the back, easing off over the spine

3

Work methodically over the back. Starting at the lower back, use reinforced hands to trace a figure-eight across the sacrum, then continue with more figure-eights up the back. Be more vigorous over fleshier areas so the receiver feels the tissues being worked. At the top, span right out over the shoulders. Finish with another large fan stroke, this time from the top to the bottom of the back.

CONTINUED ▶

BACK, SHOULDERS, AND NECK *continued*

BASIC TECHNIQUES USED
○ **Kneading, p.60**
○ **Circle strokes, p.46**
○ **Thousand hands, p.42**
○ **Criss-cross, p.48**
○ **Rocking, p.70**

Turn your focus to the lower back and spend some time working just on this area. Using your fingers and thumbs, knead deeply into the muscles on the opposite (contralateral) side of the back, warming the muscles up thoroughly in preparation for even deeper tissue work.

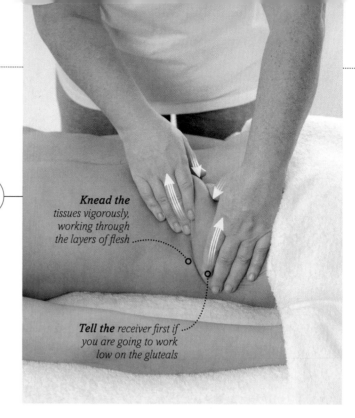

Knead the tissues vigorously, working through the layers of flesh

Tell the receiver first if you are going to work low on the gluteals

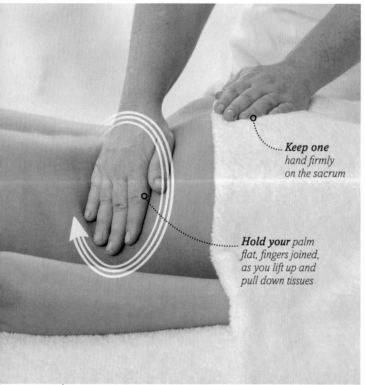

Keep one hand firmly on the sacrum

Hold your palm flat, fingers joined, as you lift up and pull down tissues

5 **Use your palm** now to apply deeper pressure to the gluteal muscles, checking the receiver is comfortable. Circle your hand very slowly, pushing into the tissues and taking care to avoid the spine.

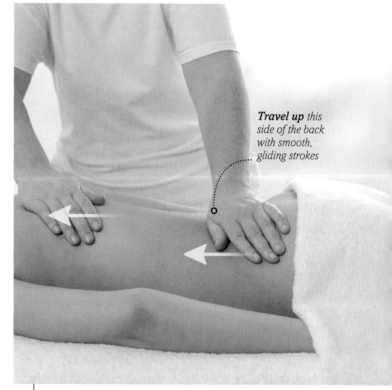

Travel up this side of the back with smooth, gliding strokes

6 **Finish this side** of the lower back with some lighter effleurage to soothe the tissues, then use thousand hands or criss-cross to travel up to and over the shoulder as you move around to the opposite side.

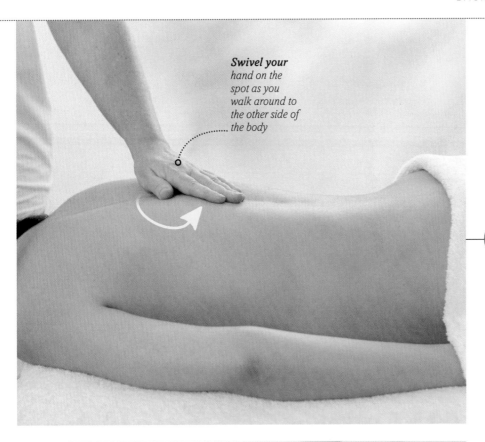

Swivel your hand on the spot as you walk around to the other side of the body

7

Keep one hand on the back to make sure you never lose contact as you move around to work on the other side of the body. This constant touch lets the receiver know where you are when they are face down so he or she is aware of what's happening at all times. Repeat all the moves on the opposite side.

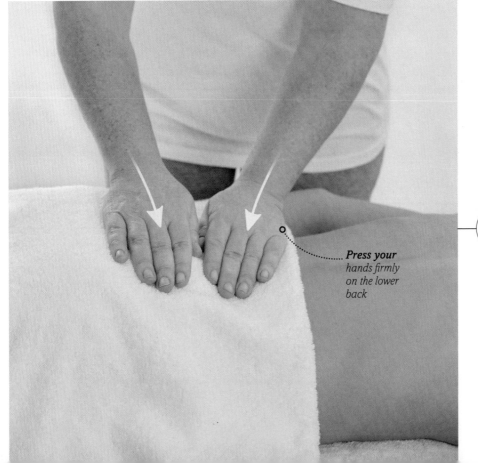

Press your hands firmly on the lower back

8

When you have finished working on the lower back, cover it with the towel. Place both hands over the towel and give the back a gentle rock. These actions keep the area warm and signal the end of your work to the lower back before you move on to the upper back and shoulders.

CONTINUED ▶

BACK, SHOULDERS, AND NECK *continued*

BASIC TECHNIQUES USED:
○ Circle strokes, p.46
○ Deep strokes, p.52
○ Static pressure, p.72

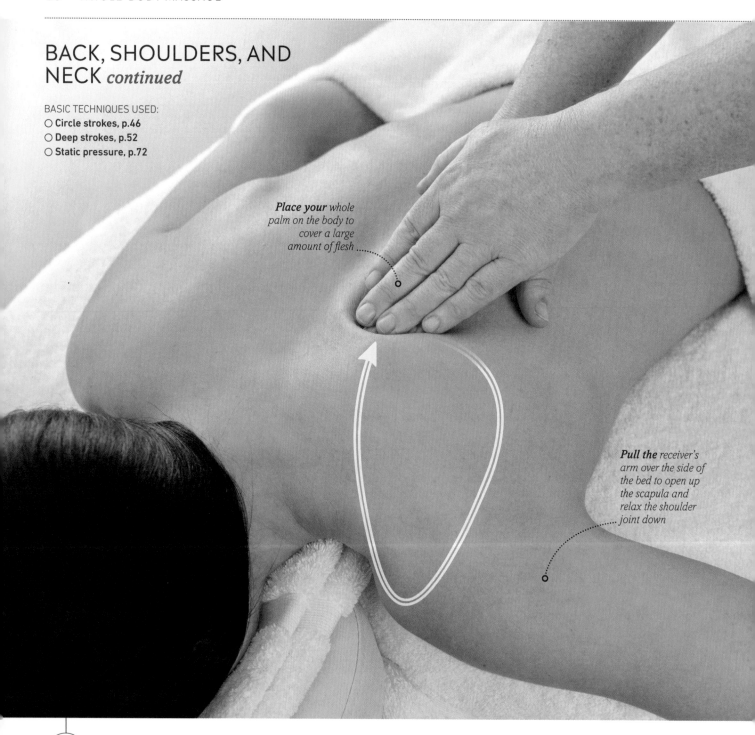

Place your whole palm on the body to cover a large amount of flesh

Pull the receiver's arm over the side of the bed to open up the scapula and relax the shoulder joint down

(9) **Moving up to the shoulders**, use reinforced hands to circle the whole of the shoulder blade. Standing on the same side as the shoulder (ipsilaterally), begin with fairly light pressure, then deepen the pressure as you continue and the tissues release. Do several rotations.

"Build pressure gradually, sensing the release of the tissues as you work over an area."

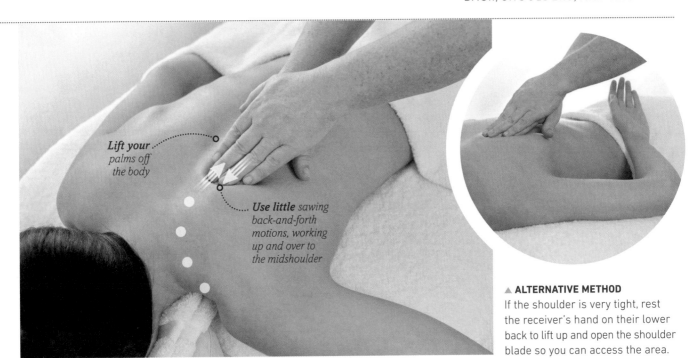

Lift your palms off the body

Use little sawing back-and-forth motions, working up and over to the midshoulder

▲ **ALTERNATIVE METHOD**
If the shoulder is very tight, rest the receiver's hand on their lower back to lift up and open the shoulder blade so you can access the area.

10   **Use just reinforced fingers** to massage more deeply, working across and down into the tissues in a back-and-forth action. Check the receiver's comfort and take care when you reach the nerves at the top of the back. Finish with another whole-hand circle to soothe the tissues.

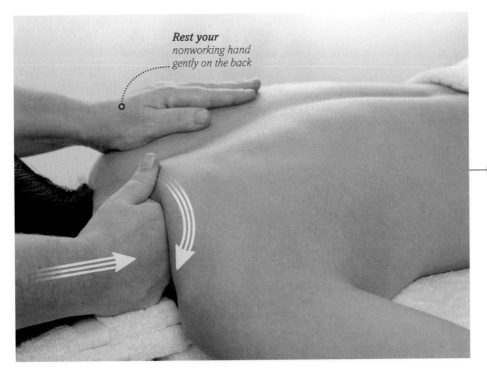

Rest your nonworking hand gently on the back

11   **Stand at the head** of the table to start work on the neck. Hold your hand in a fairly tight fist, then press down into the curve of the neck. Push forward deeply into the flesh, then fan your fist out to midshoulder, taking care to work very slowly while applying this deeper pressure. Repeat two or three times.

CONTINUED ▶

BACK, SHOULDERS, AND NECK *continued*

BASIC TECHNIQUES USED
○ **Kneading, p.60**
○ **Circle strokes, p.46**
○ **Slide and glide, p.44**
○ **Stretches, p.74**

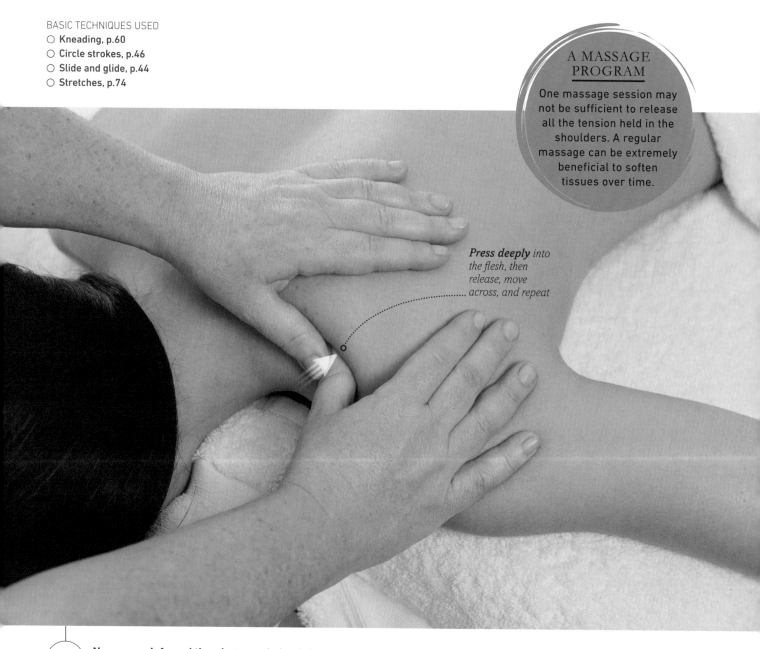

Press deeply into the flesh, then release, move across, and repeat

A MASSAGE PROGRAM

One massage session may not be sufficient to release all the tension held in the shoulders. A regular massage can be extremely beneficial to soften tissues over time.

(12) **Now use reinforced thumbs** to work deeply into the tissues. Start at the base of the head, then move down the neck around the scapula. Squat and put your body weight into the move to protect your thumbs. (You can also apply pressure to the working thumb with the palm of your other hand.) If the tissues are very tight, work down the rhomboid on the side of the spine.

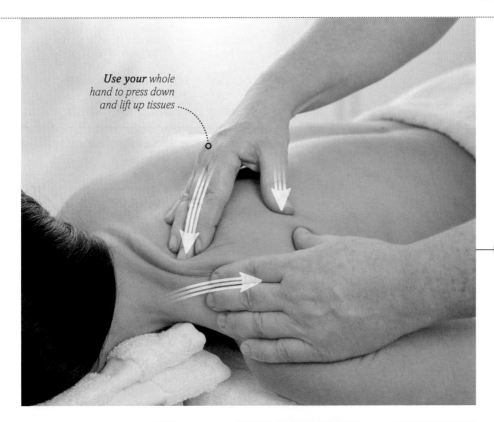

Use your whole hand to press down and lift up tissues

To soothe the tissues after the deeper pressure, knead over the shoulder. If, at this point, the tissues still feel tense, try doing a little more deep tissue work to loosen them. Finish with another reinforced hand circle, then put the arm back on the bed.

⟨13⟩

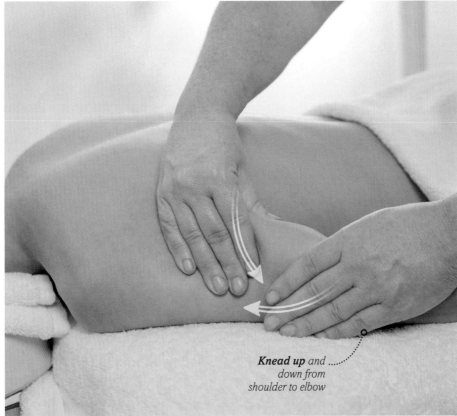

Knead up and down from shoulder to elbow

Lightly effleurage the upper arm, then follow with some kneading. This connects the shoulder with the triceps and ensures that you don't miss the very edge of the shoulder. Repeat everything on the opposite shoulder and arm. Finish the back by effleuraging all over and then gently stretching the neck. Cover the back with a towel and stroke the shoulders. Place your hands on the back to signal the end of the massage to this area.

⟨14⟩

BACK OF THE LEGS

The legs can become heavy and sluggish when tired and can carry everyday strain. Massaging the legs can be both relaxing and energizing for the receiver and has a positive impact on the whole body. Check if the lower back feels pinched—in which case, it can be helpful to separate the legs a little. Also, if there is a gap beneath the ankles, place a rolled-up towel under them for support.

BASIC TECHNIQUES USED
○ **Thousand hands, p.42**
○ **Slide and glide, p.44**
○ **Wringing, p.56**
○ **Deep strokes, p.52**
○ **Kneading, p.60**

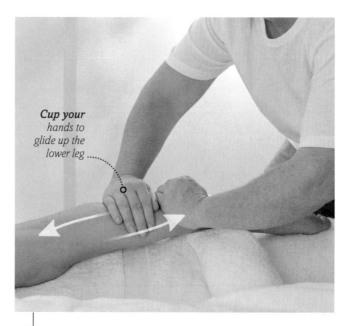

Cup your hands to glide up the lower leg

1 **Effleurage up and down** the whole leg, using a cupping action on the calf and a thousand hands on the thigh, keeping pressure light over the knee. This warms the tissues, and the large, gliding strokes are extremely soothing.

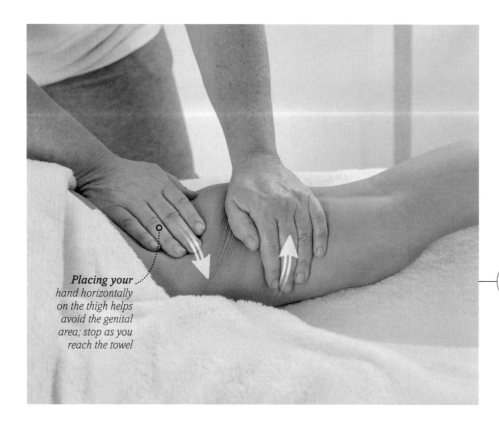

Placing your hand horizontally on the thigh helps avoid the genital area; stop as you reach the towel

PREVENT BLOCKAGES

Petrissage the thigh before the calf. This drains lymphatic waste in the upper leg first, eliminating blockages and ensuring that waste can drain freely from the lower leg.

2 **Once you have warmed up** the thigh tissues with some lighter effleurage, wring over the back of the thigh to release tension and help flush out waste. Follow this with other petrissage techniques.

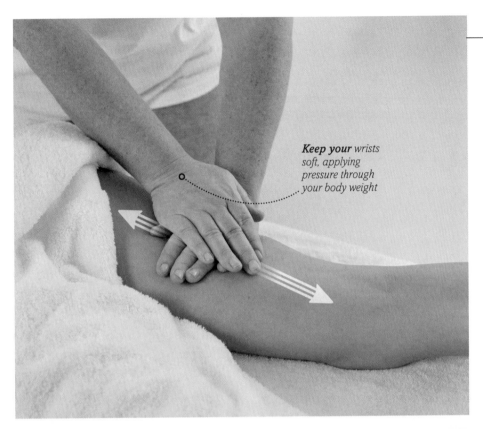

Keep your wrists *soft, applying pressure through your body weight*

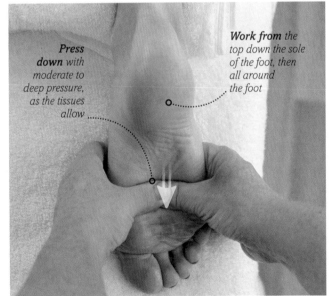

③

Now use reinforced hands to work deeply into the fleshy thigh. Start at the top in the gluteal muscles, stop before the knee, then turn and travel back, working slowly and carefully. Reinforced hands can also be used on the calf, but only in one direction here, from the ankle to the knee.

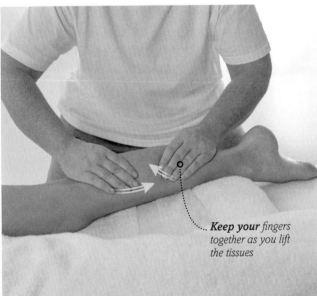

Keep your fingers *together as you lift the tissues*

Press down with *moderate to deep pressure, as the tissues allow*

Work from the top down the sole of the foot, then all around the foot

④ Petrissage the lower leg, squatting down low and moving your body from side to side to direct the action as you knead up and down the fleshy muscle, from above the ankle to just below the back of the knee.

⑤ Finish on the foot, checking first if the receiver is happy for this to be touched. Use reinforced thumbs to relax tissues, working carefully in areas of resistance. Repeat everything on the opposite leg.

FRONT OF THE FEET AND LEGS

Help the receiver to turn (see p.81) to lie on their back—supine—as you start work on the front of the body. Once turned, make sure the receiver is comfortable, placing a rolled towel, bolster, or pillow under the knees for support and positioning towels for warmth and modesty. Ask the receiver to take a few deep breaths in and out while you place your hands on the legs in a grounding hold. Working on the front of the legs and feet first completes work to this part of the body before you move up, finishing your massage on the upper body.

BASIC TECHNIQUES USED
○ **Slide and glide, p.44**
○ **Thousand hands, p.42**
○ **Wringing, p.56**
○ **Kneading, p.60**
○ **Deep stroke, p.52**

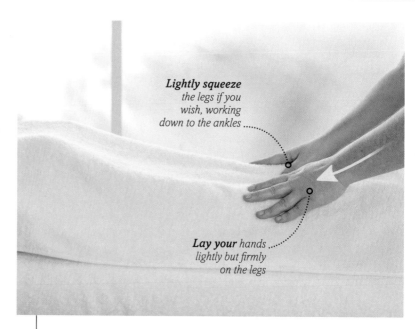

Lightly squeeze the legs if you wish, working down to the ankles

Lay your hands lightly but firmly on the legs

1 **Rest your hands** on the legs over the towel, giving the receiver time to calm their breathing after turning and allowing yourself a moment to refocus before you massage the front of the body.

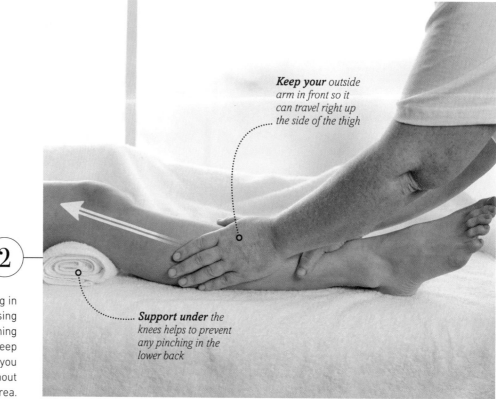

Keep your outside arm in front so it can travel right up the side of the thigh

2 **Effleurage up** the whole leg in long, sweeping strokes, using moderate pressure and lightening pressure over the kneecap. Keep your hand in a "V" shape so you can work up the entire leg without going near the genital area.

Support under the knees helps to prevent any pinching in the lower back

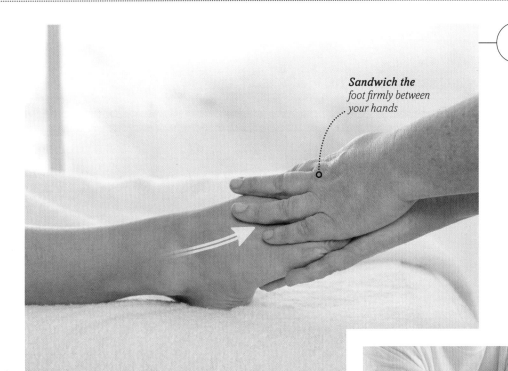

Sandwich the foot firmly between your hands

(3)

Glide back down the leg and finish by holding the foot between both hands. Glide your hands right to the end of the foot and gently stretch the foot out. Hold the foot for a moment before sliding your hands off.

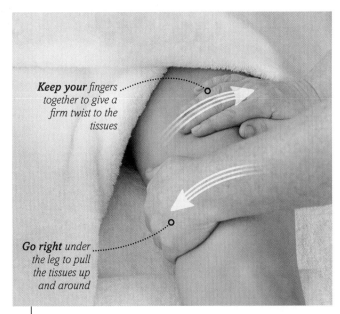

Keep your fingers together to give a firm twist to the tissues

Go right under the leg to pull the tissues up and around

Keep your hands and wrists straight, lunging in to lean into the move with your body weight

Put your outside hand on the thigh, your inside hand on top

(4) **Move to the thigh.** Start with some energetic thousand hands effleurage. Follow with deeper petrissage, first wringing over this fleshy area, as shown above, then doing some vigorous kneading to warm the tissues and tone the muscles.

(5) **Use reinforced hands** to apply deeper pressure along the thigh above the knee. Move gently at first into the tissues, pressing along the tissues—not straight down, which could damage them. Finish off the thigh with some soothing effleurage.

CONTINUED ▶

FRONT OF THE FEET AND LEGS *continued*

BASIC TECHNIQUES USED
○ Static pressure, p.72
○ Kneading, p.60
○ Circle strokes, p.46
○ Stretches, p.74

"Move your body rhythmically side to side when facing the body to work up and down a limb."

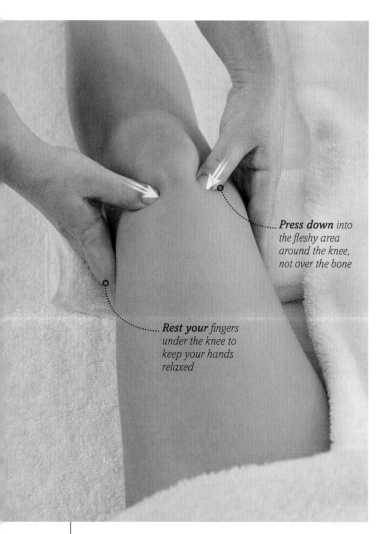

Press down into the fleshy area around the knee, not over the bone

Rest your fingers under the knee to keep your hands relaxed

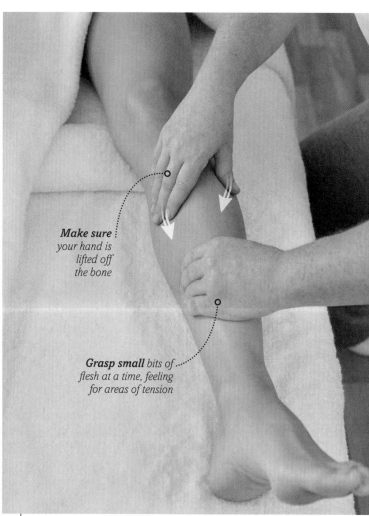

Make sure your hand is lifted off the bone

Grasp small bits of flesh at a time, feeling for areas of tension

(6) **Work gently** around—not over—the knee, applying static pressure with your thumbs to work into pressure points around the knee, from top to bottom. Glide back up or work back up over the pressure points.

(7) **Effleurage the calf**, then knead more deeply into the fleshy areas on either side of the bone. Travel up and down, moving your body side to side to get a good rhythm. Finish with some soothing effleurage.

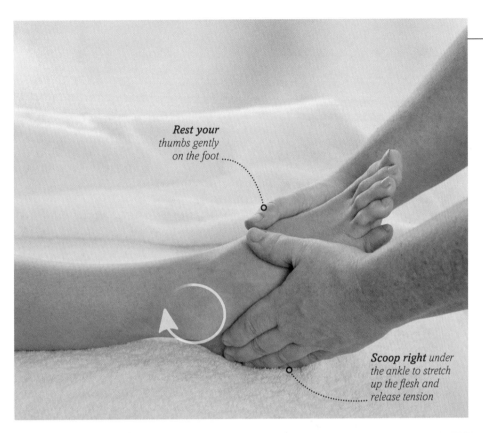

Rest your thumbs gently on the foot

Scoop right under the ankle to stretch up the flesh and release tension

8

Move down to the foot—an area where tension is often held—to warm the tissues with some relaxing effleurage. Circle your fingers around the ankle bones, applying moderate pressure and working simultaneously on either side of the foot to soothe and relax tissues.

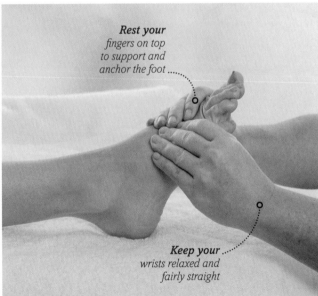

Rest your fingers on top to support and anchor the foot

Keep your wrists relaxed and fairly straight

9 **Knead the sole** of the foot with your thumbs, working deeply into tissues to release tension in this hardworking area. Knead from the bottom to the top, then back down in an elongated circle.

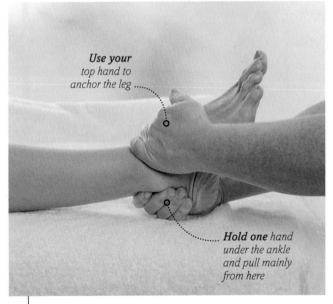

Use your top hand to anchor the leg

Hold one hand under the ankle and pull mainly from here

10 **Effleurage up and down** the leg and finish with a whole leg stretch. In a lunge, lean your body weight back to get a nice pull on the leg, releasing tension in the hips. Repeat everything on the opposite leg.

ABDOMEN

This important area, which houses several internal organs, can feel vulnerable to touch, so check first that the receiver is happy for you to work on the abdomen. If he or she is comfortable being touched here, this will be an extremely nurturing and calming part of their massage, as you work on the energy center of the body. The key to abdominal massage is to go very slowly and gently, building pressure and expanding over the area gradually.

BASIC TECHNIQUES USED
○ **Circle strokes, p.46**
○ **Slide and glide, p.44**

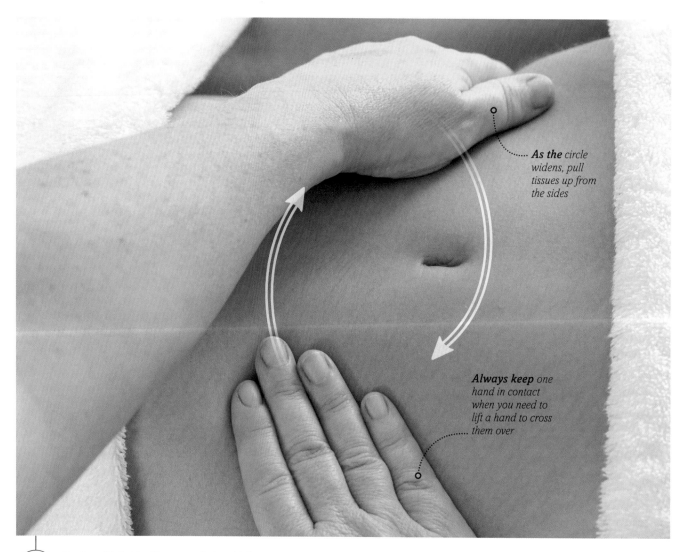

As the circle widens, pull tissues up from the sides

Always keep one hand in contact when you need to lift a hand to cross them over

(1) **Begin with** light effleurage circles. Make small, slow clockwise circles with both hands, starting bottom right to follow the path of the intestines. Gradually widen the circle and build pressure.

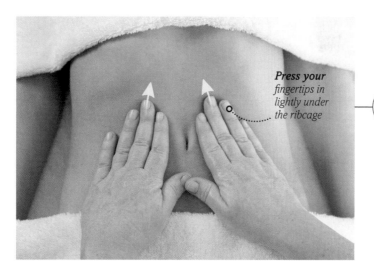

Press your *fingertips in* *lightly under* *the ribcage*

2

Follow circling with the stretching and pulling sequence shown here and continued in steps 3 and 4. These three steps should be carried out in one flowing movement. First, place both hands on either side of the belly button, below the ribcage.

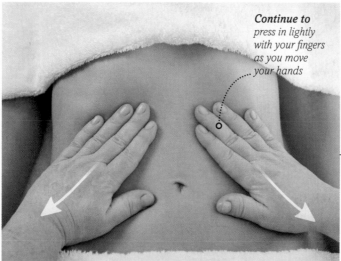

Continue to *press in lightly* *with your fingers* *as you move* *your hands*

3

From the starting position in step 2, sweep your palms outward in opposite directions over the ribs, right down to the sides of the body.

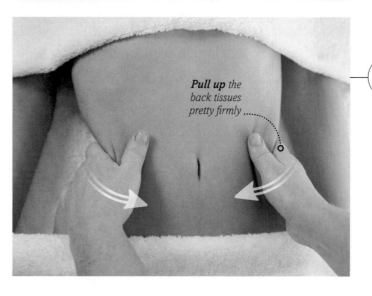

Pull up *the* *back tissues* *pretty firmly*

4

As you sweep your hands down, hook them under the body—avoiding the spine—and gather up the muscle, then scoop them back up, pulling the muscle up, too. This sequence releases tension in both the abdomen and the lower back as muscles connected to the pelvic area are worked on and nerves on the back are soothed.

HANDS AND ARMS

Chronic tension from the shoulders can often be felt in the hands and arms, so it's important not to neglect this part of the body and to treat the hands and arms as an extension of the shoulders. Our hands also do a great deal of work, much of it repetitive, and both the hands and arms can hold tension, so massage is extremely beneficial here.

BASIC TECHNIQUES USED
○ **Shaking, p.68**
○ **Slide and glide, p.44**
○ **Kneading, p.60**

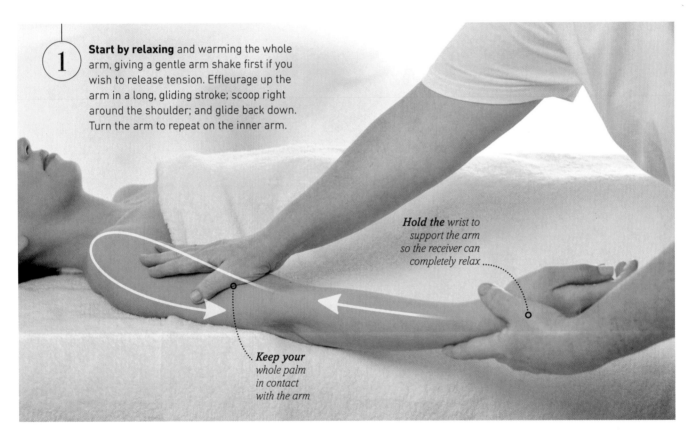

1 **Start by relaxing** and warming the whole arm, giving a gentle arm shake first if you wish to release tension. Effleurage up the arm in a long, gliding stroke; scoop right around the shoulder; and glide back down. Turn the arm to repeat on the inner arm.

Hold the wrist to support the arm so the receiver can completely relax

Keep your whole palm in contact with the arm

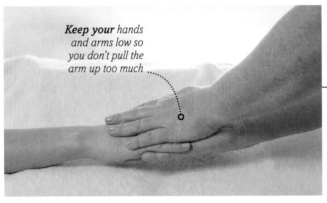

Keep your hands and arms low so you don't pull the arm up too much

2 **Sandwich the hand** between your hands, holding it firmly but without pressing, then lean back, giving a gentle pull to the hand to lengthen and relax the whole limb.

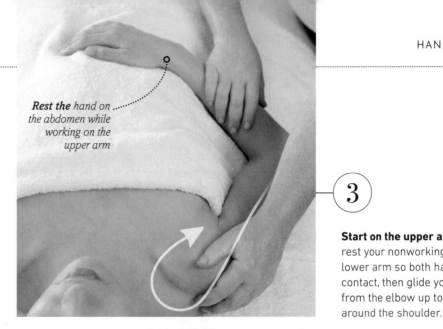

Rest the hand on
the abdomen while
working on the
upper arm

3

Start on the upper arm. Lightly rest your nonworking hand on the lower arm so both hands are in contact, then glide your other hand from the elbow up to the neck and around the shoulder.

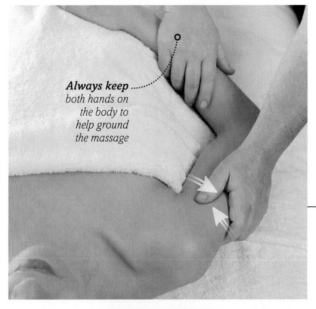

Always keep
both hands on
the body to
help ground
the massage

4

In a fluid action, travel back down the upper arm using one-handed kneading to work into the fleshy muscle here.

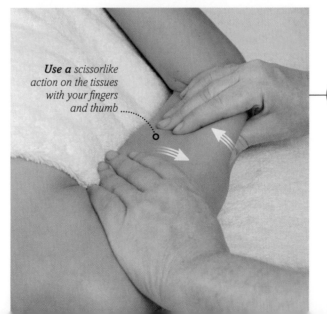

Use a scissorlike
action on the tissues
with your fingers
and thumb

5

Stand side-on to the arm in a squat position and use both hands to knead and glide simultaneously up and down the biceps, releasing tension in this muscle. Move your body from side to side to direct your action up and down the upper arm.

CONTINUED ▶

HANDS AND ARMS
continued

BASIC TECHNIQUES USED
○ **Slide and glide, p.44**
○ **Deep strokes, p.52**
○ **Kneading, p.60**

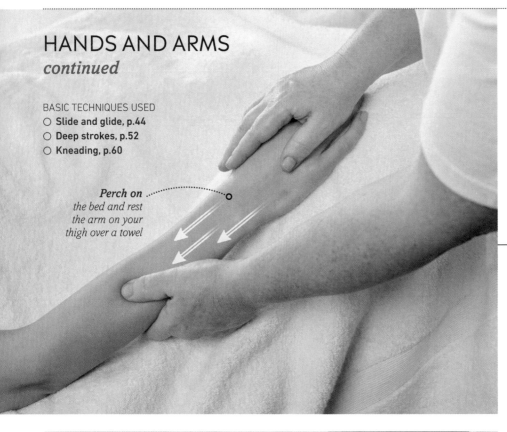

Perch on the bed and rest the arm on your thigh over a towel

6

Glide up the lower arm with your thumb, working deeply into the muscle. Start at the midpoint above the wrist and glide up to the elbow. Repeat this glide on the outer and inner edges of the arm to work all of the lower arm muscles. Finish with some soothing effleurage.

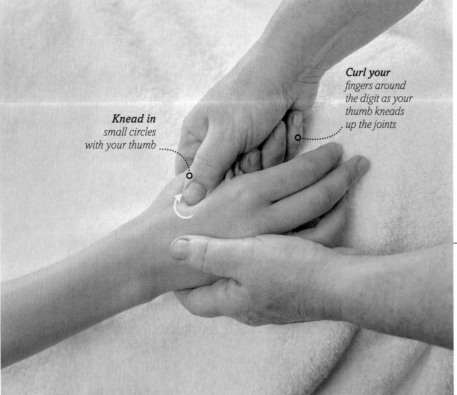

Knead in small circles with your thumb

Curl your fingers around the digit as your thumb kneads up the joints

7

Work on each finger in turn, beginning with the thumb. Hold the hand to support it, then with your other hand, start at the bottom of the joint and knead all the way up toward the tip, giving a gentle squeeze at the tip to finish.

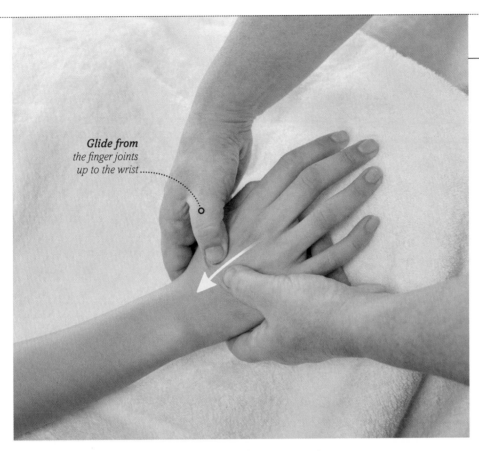

Glide from
the finger joints
up to the wrist ....

(8)

Relax the front of the hand with some gentle effleurage. Resting the heel of the hand in your palms, glide your thumbs between the bones of each finger in turn.

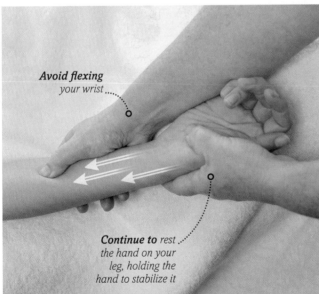

Avoid flexing
your wrist ....

Continue to rest
the hand on your
leg, holding the
hand to stabilize it

(9) **Turn the arm around** to work on the inner arm with the same thumb-gliding technique you used on the front of the arm and applying the same amount of pressure to the inner arm.

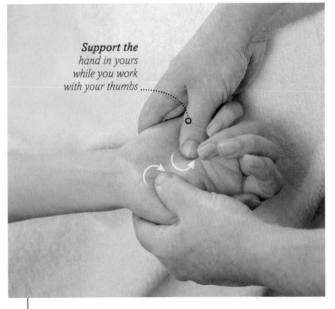

Support the
hand in yours
while you work
with your thumbs ....

(10) **Knead the palm** with your thumbs to ease residual tension. When you have finished on the hand, effleurage the arm again, sandwich the hand, and gently glide your hands off. Put the arm back under the towel, then repeat all the steps on the other arm.

UPPER CHEST, SHOULDERS, AND NECK

BASIC TECHNIQUES USED
- **Slide and glide, p.44**
- **Stretches, p.74**

The upper chest, shoulders, and neck can often be tight due to factors such as poor posture or excessive keyboard work hunching the shoulders forward. The sequence below, done in one fluid move, opens up the chest and releases tension and should always form part of your whole-body sequence. If the chin is higher than the forehead, raise the head on a folded towel or blanket.

Lay your palms flat, squatting low to avoid flexing your wrists

Take care not to press down on the breast tissue on women (You can work farther down into the pectorals on men)

NATURAL FLOW

This sequence follows on naturally from the arms as you are circling around the shoulder joint, this time from a different angle, working with the contours of the body.

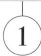

Place your hands at the top of the chest in the center. This introduces touch to the upper chest and prepares it for some warming effleurage.

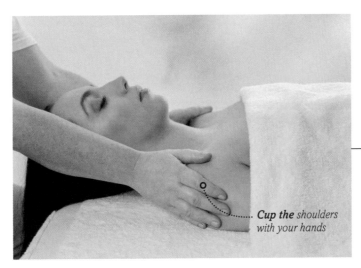

Cup the shoulders *with your hands*

(2)

Sweep your hands out over the shoulders, pressing down on the shoulders briefly to open up the chest area.

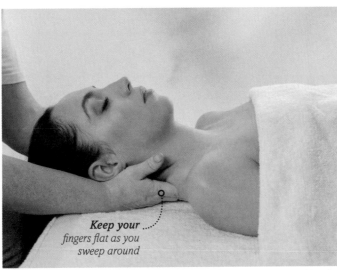

Keep your fingers flat as you sweep around

(3)

Scoop your hands right under the shoulders, then sweep them up under the base of the neck.

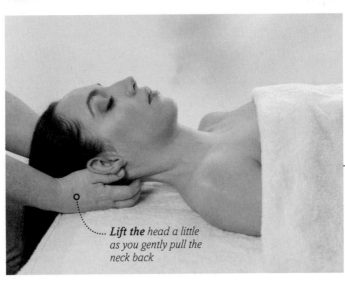

Lift the head a little as you gently pull the neck back

(4)

Now curl your fingers a little and pull back the flesh under the neck, giving the neck a gentle stretch as you do so to finish.

NECK

Take great care when working on the neck, especially when turning the head or stretching the neck muscles. Before starting the sequence below, center the head, then cup the ears with your hands when turning the head to either side. Do this slowly and calmly and never force a stretch in the neck.

BASIC TECHNIQUES USED
○ **Rotations, p.76**
○ **Stretches, p.74**
○ **Slide and glide, p.44**
○ **Kneading, p.60**

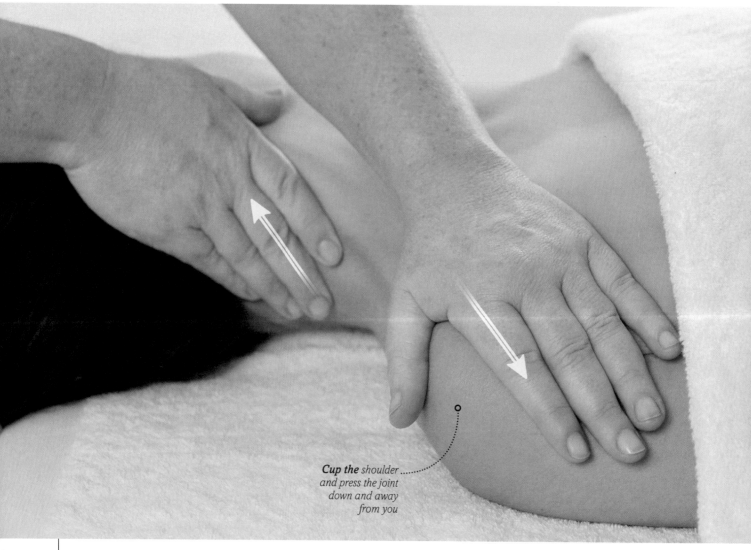

Cup the shoulder *and press the joint down and away from you*

① **Start working on the neck** with a gentle stretch. Place your far hand on the opposite shoulder and cradle the base of the head with your other hand. Keeping the neck anchored, gently push the shoulder joint away to create a stretch in the neck.

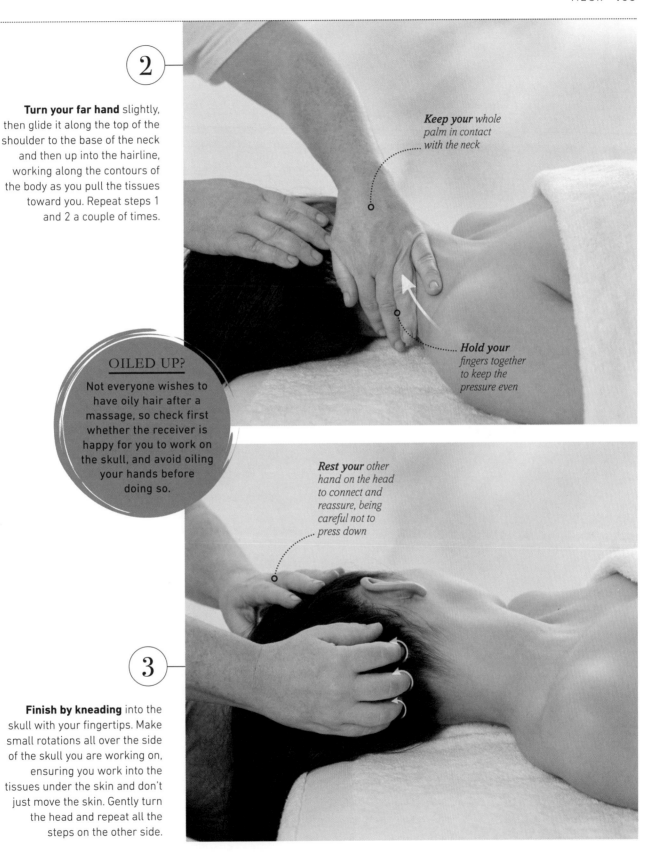

2

Turn your far hand slightly, then glide it along the top of the shoulder to the base of the neck and then up into the hairline, working along the contours of the body as you pull the tissues toward you. Repeat steps 1 and 2 a couple of times.

Keep your whole palm in contact with the neck

Hold your fingers together to keep the pressure even

OILED UP?

Not everyone wishes to have oily hair after a massage, so check first whether the receiver is happy for you to work on the skull, and avoid oiling your hands before doing so.

Rest your other hand on the head to connect and reassure, being careful not to press down

3

Finish by kneading into the skull with your fingertips. Make small rotations all over the side of the skull you are working on, ensuring you work into the tissues under the skin and don't just move the skin. Gently turn the head and repeat all the steps on the other side.

FACE AND HEAD

Massaging around the face and head is a deeply relaxing way to finish your whole-body sequence. The aim here is to relax the facial muscles and help the jaw muscles, which are often clenched, to let go of tension. If you wish, once you have completed this final part of the body, feather over the sides of the torso (avoiding the breast and genital area) and the legs over the towel, lift the towel to stroke the feet and gently pull the ankles, then cover the feet again and place your hands on them.

BASIC TECHNIQUES USED
○ **Circle stroke, p.46**
○ **Kneading, p.60**
○ **Stretches, p.74**

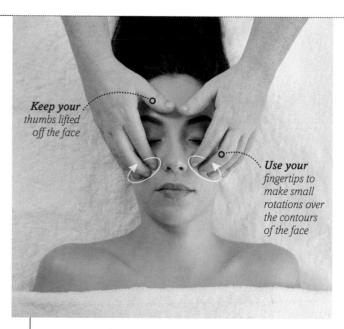

Keep your thumbs lifted off the face

Use your fingertips to make small rotations over the contours of the face

1 **Circle over** the face. Work from the center outward, first on the forehead, then from the nose, over the jawline, to the chin. Repeat, going deeper on the jaw this time to relieve tension here.

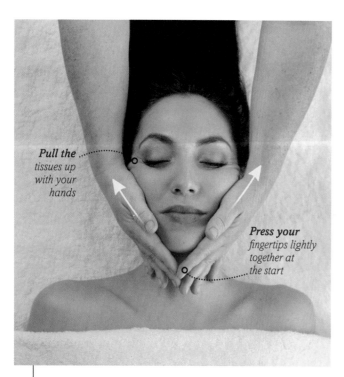

Pull the tissues up with your hands

Press your fingertips lightly together at the start

2 **Cup the chin**. Sweep along the jaw, move up, sweep out from the nose, and sweep up the sides. Finish by kneading the skull, pressing your fingers in to move the tissues.

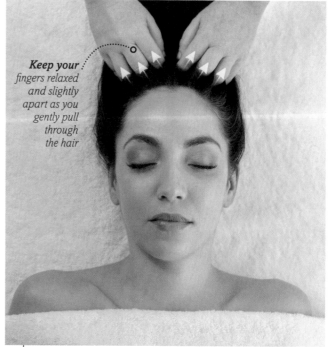

Keep your fingers relaxed and slightly apart as you gently pull through the hair

3 **Using just the tips** of your fingers, rake slowly back through the hair, pulling gently to create a deeply relaxing effect.

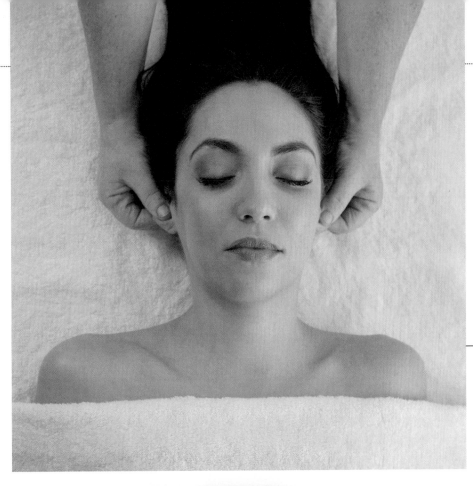

④

Knead the fleshy parts of the ears between your index finger and thumb, working on acupressure points to reawaken and energize the receiver as the massage comes to a close.

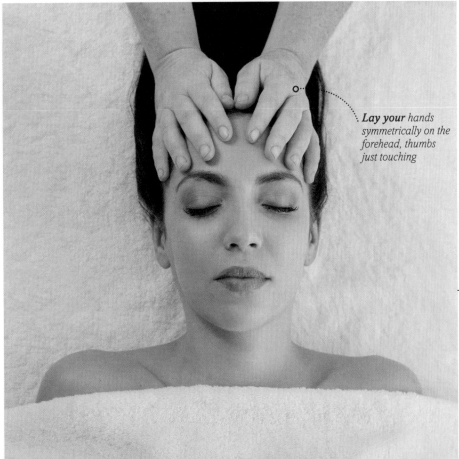

Lay your hands symmetrically on the forehead, thumbs just touching

⑤

To signal the end of work to the face and head, place your hands on the forehead, cupping the skull. Gently pull the skin if you wish to give a sense of release.

SPECIALTIES

Once basic massage techniques are mastered, practitioners may wish to develop their practice to specialize in one or more areas. The following pages provide a brief introduction to some of the main massage specialties that can be pursued with further training, including Western-based practices that work on the principle of softening tissues and improving mobility; practices that work on the principle of correcting the subtle energy flow within the body, such as Ayurveda; and disciplines that work on a specific part of the body, such as reflexology. For each specialty, core principles or belief systems are explained and photographs of techniques illustrate some of the key elements of the practice.

KEY

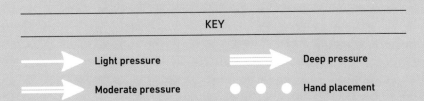

Light pressure

Deep pressure

Moderate pressure

Hand placement

ESSENCE	TECHNIQUES	BENEFITS
Increases local blood and lymph circulation; eases adhesions between fibers.	A set of techniques is used to achieve different effects and pressures.	Helps reduce muscular pain and tension and emotional stress.

HOW DOES SWEDISH MASSAGE WORK?

During a Swedish massage, the group of basic techniques that Mezger developed are used to manipulate soft tissues in the body. Different techniques are combined and/or adapted to meet the needs of each individual. One of the key characteristics of Swedish massage is that the strokes are carried out in a smooth, flowing rhythm and the amount of pressure is adapted to suit the receiver's own preference and the area or complaint that is being treated.

The massage treatments take place on a massage couch using just a small amount of oil so that the practitioner's hands are able to move smoothly and comfortably over the skin while still ensuring that there is sufficient friction from strokes for the deeper tissue structures to be manipulated.

The aims of Swedish massage are to reduce muscular tension throughout the body by increasing the local circulation of blood and lymphatic fluids; to stretch muscle fibers; and to reduce adhesions, or stickiness, in scar tissues to help improve the appearance of scars. Swedish massage also stimulates the peripheral nervous system (see p.20), which in turn helps encourage both physical and emotional relaxation.

SPECIALTIES

SWEDISH MASSAGE

Swedish, or classical, massage is one of the most recognized types of massage in the West. Its origins lie in traditional massage techniques practiced in Europe that were formalized in the 1800s into groups of therapeutic techniques by a Dutch doctor named Johann Georg Mezger. The groups he developed comprise effleurage (stroking), petrissage (kneading), tapotement (percussion or tapping), and vibration (shaking and rocking).

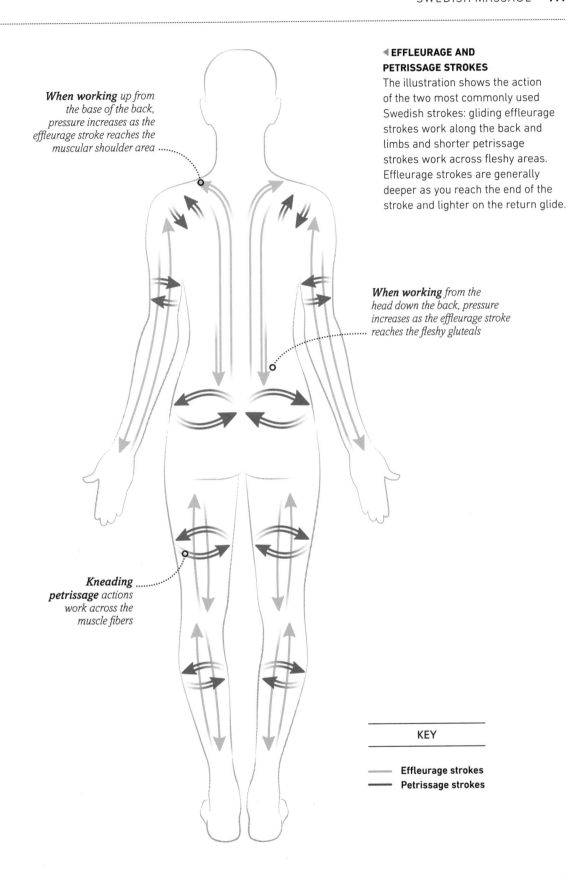

When working up from the base of the back, pressure increases as the effleurage stroke reaches the muscular shoulder area

◀ EFFLEURAGE AND PETRISSAGE STROKES
The illustration shows the action of the two most commonly used Swedish strokes: gliding effleurage strokes work along the back and limbs and shorter petrissage strokes work across fleshy areas. Effleurage strokes are generally deeper as you reach the end of the stroke and lighter on the return glide.

When working from the head down the back, pressure increases as the effleurage stroke reaches the fleshy gluteals

Kneading petrissage actions work across the muscle fibers

KEY

— Effleurage strokes
— Petrissage strokes

SWEDISH MASSAGE

Swedish massage is characterized by rhythmic, flowing strokes, using a little oil to help hands glide over skin. The effleurage, petrissage, and percussive strokes shown here are the most commonly used; other techniques include vibration, static and other pressures, and rotations. The repetitive actions of some of the movements can strain the fingers and especially the thumbs, so adaptations can be made to protect them.

BASIC TECHNIQUES USED:
- ○ **Effleurage, p.40**
- ○ **Petrissage, p.56**
- ○ **Percussion, p.64**
- ○ **Vibrations, p.68**
- ○ **Pressure, p.72**
- ○ **Passive movements, p.74**

| EFFLEURAGE

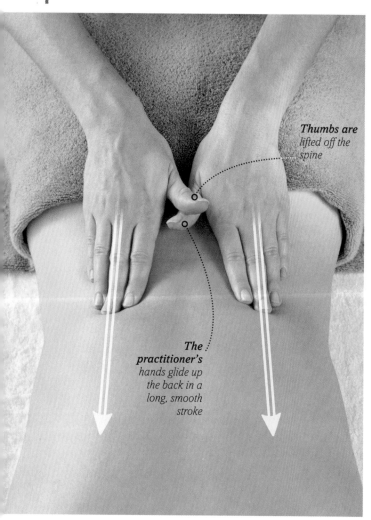

Thumbs are lifted off the spine

The practitioner's hands glide up the back in a long, smooth stroke

▲ **Long, gliding effleurage strokes** work over the body in a circular pattern as the practitioner's hands glide away, return, then repeat a stroke. "Sticky" areas may be felt where there are adhesions in tissues, which the practitioner can return to.

| PETRISSAGE

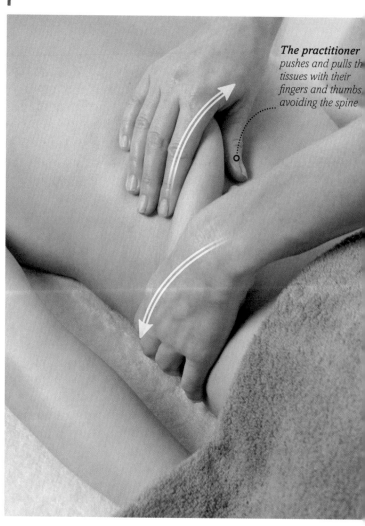

The practitioner pushes and pulls the tissues with their fingers and thumbs avoiding the spine

▲ **Techniques such as wringing**, kneading, knuckling, and skin rolling are done after effleurage has warmed up the tissues. These more vigorous techniques work along muscle fibers into the deeper layers or muscles.

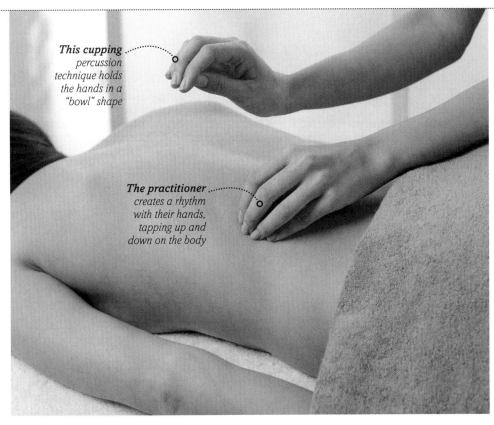

This cupping percussion technique holds the hands in a "bowl" shape

The practitioner creates a rhythm with their hands, tapping up and down on the body

— PERCUSSION

◀ **Also called "tapotement,"** these are lively actions with a steady, staccato rhythm that are used to reenergize the receiver or to break up areas of congestion.

▌ PROTECTING THE THUMBS

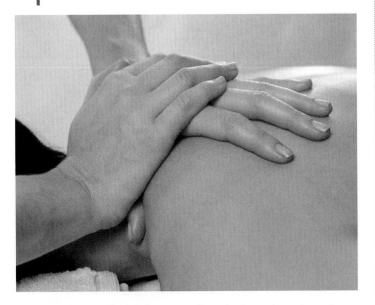

▲ **Working on knotted areas** such as the trapezius, where deep pressure may be applied, can strain thumbs. The practitioner can protect their thumb by using their other hand to apply pressure so the thumb can sink into tissues without straining itself.

▌ SUPPORTING THE FINGERS

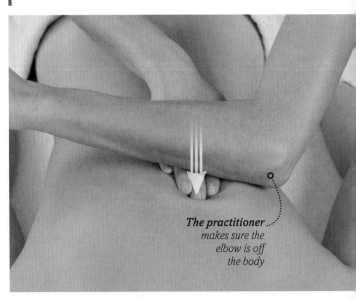

The practitioner makes sure the elbow is off the body

▲ **The forearm can be used** to support all of the fingers when working along a long expanse such as the back or the thigh. The support of the forearm means the bottom hand can work deeply into the tissues without putting strain on its fingers.

KEY FACTS

ESSENCE	TECHNIQUES	BENEFITS
Aims to address areas of tightness caused by physical and emotional stress.	Various, including work on deeper musculoskeletal structures.	Reduces chronic pain and restrictions where fascia has tightened.

HOW DOES DEEP TISSUE MASSAGE WORK?

Deep tissue massage helps "organize" and restore elasticity to fascia—the web of connective tissue that surrounds all of the body's structures—when this has shortened or tightened due to trauma, inflammation, or repetitive movement. This in turn relieves the pain caused by chronic muscle tension and myofascial (the fascia surrounding muscles) restrictions, which cause structures in the body to become misaligned. Deep tissue massage also boosts local blood and lymph circulation, improving the health of congested muscles, and can provide relief from emotional stress.

Deep tissue treatments are usually carried out on a massage couch, which may need to be lowered to allow the practitioner to lean in (see p.116). Some preliminary Swedish massage techniques are given to relax the body first and soften tissues in the area to be treated. Deep tissue work is then applied to local areas that are causing a particular issue rather than over the entire body, although it can be incorporated into a full-body massage. The knuckles, heel of the hand, elbow, and forearm can all be used—along with the movement of the practitioner's body weight— to adjust pressure, and strokes are carried out parallel to or across the direction of the muscle fibers. The careful, slow approach means that the practitioner can work well within the receiver's pain threshold.

SPECIALTIES

DEEP TISSUE MASSAGE

Deep tissue massage is usually characterized by firm, slow strokes that allow the therapist to sink into deeper layers of muscle and connective tissue. Its origins are hard to pin down, but there have been a number of practitioners who have developed different techniques in the more recent history of massage that have been incorporated into deep tissue massage treatments today. Deep tissue massage aims to improve tissue and joint movement, reduce chronic pain, and relax.

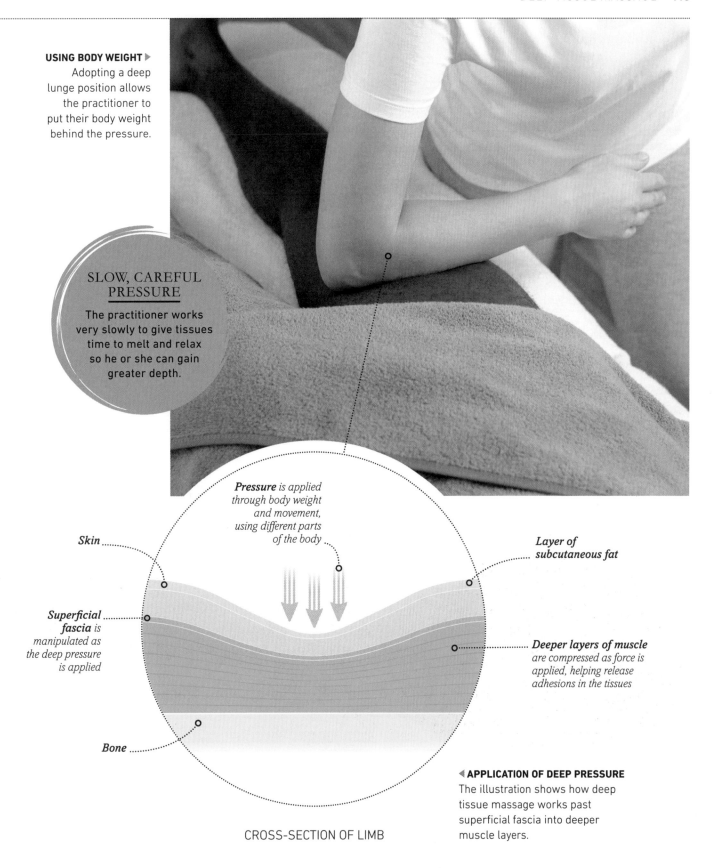

USING BODY WEIGHT ▷
Adopting a deep lunge position allows the practitioner to put their body weight behind the pressure.

SLOW, CAREFUL
PRESSURE

The practitioner works very slowly to give tissues time to melt and relax so he or she can gain greater depth.

Pressure is applied through body weight and movement, using different parts of the body

Skin

Layer of subcutaneous fat

Superficial fascia is manipulated as the deep pressure is applied

Deeper layers of muscle are compressed as force is applied, helping release adhesions in the tissues

Bone

CROSS-SECTION OF LIMB

◀ APPLICATION OF DEEP PRESSURE
The illustration shows how deep tissue massage works past superficial fascia into deeper muscle layers.

DEEP TISSUE MASSAGE

In deep tissue work, the practitioner uses their own body weight to apply pressure and sink into deeper muscle layers and connective tissues, positioning the bed and their body to avoid strain. As well as the forearm, the elbow, knuckles, or heel of the hand can be used, while minimal oil gives movement without slippage. Other Swedish techniques are carried out first to soften and prep the area.

BASIC TECHNIQUES USED
○ **Deep strokes, p.52**
○ **Effleurage strokes, p.40**
○ **Petrissage strokes, p.56**
○ **Static pressure, p.72**

Keeping the wrist limp and relaxed avoids transferring tension to the forearm

The practitioner keeps the forearm flat, ensuring that the elbow is not pressing into flesh

▌ DEEP TISSUE STROKES

▲ **To work deeply** into tissues in a gliding action, the practitioner needs to lunge low and lean right into the body, lowering the bed sufficiently to use body weight effectively. The forearm is ideal for moving very slowly over large areas of muscle, such as the trapezius and thighs.

DEEP STATIC PRESSURE

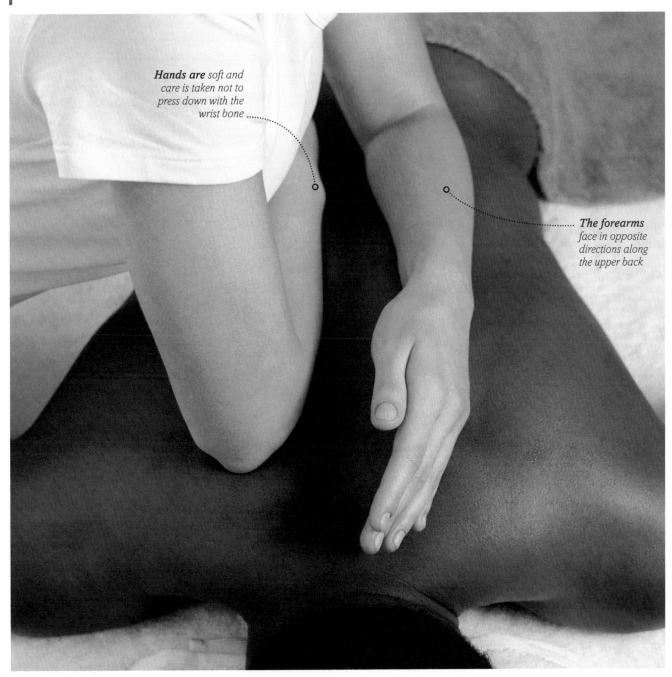

Hands are soft and care is taken not to press down with the wrist bone

The forearms face in opposite directions along the upper back

▲ **To apply deep pressure** in one place, the practitioner leans over the body, squatting if needed. Both forearms can be used to apply pressure simultaneously on either side of the spine, leaning in and down, releasing, and repeating as needed. The bed may need lowering even farther here to enable the practitioner to lean right over the body.

KEY FACTS

ESSENCE	TECHNIQUES	BENEFITS
A standalone treatment for stress, or done in conjunction with psychotherapy.	Massage is done while listening to the gut to assess how effective a treatment is.	Helps restore balance to the mind, body, and energy systems.

SPECIALTIES

BIODYNAMIC MASSAGE

Biodynamic massage was developed by psychologist Gerda Boyesen in the 1960s after she became interested in the effect of touch and massage on people with mental illness. Biodynamic psychology is based on the belief that there is a connection between the mind, body, and spirit. The massage practice developed as a branch of this, integrating the principles of psychotherapy with massage to create a form of body psychotherapy.

HOW DOES BIODYNAMIC MASSAGE WORK?

Biodynamic massage can be carried out directly on the skin or through clothing. It works on the basis that the brain and gut affect each other, so by listening to the gut, the practitioner can detect the body's unconscious response to touch. Audible gut activity is viewed as a sign of relaxation, indicating that the body feels emotionally safe. To achieve this, an electronic stethoscope is placed on the body to observe the sounds of the gut while a variety of techniques is used.

The practitioner uses the techniques that are most suited to how the person is feeling. Techniques include stretching, connective tissue work, and light energetic touch. Sometimes a person's aura, or energy field, will be worked on to balance energy around the body. Other specialized techniques use the breath to release trapped nervous reactions, such as a "frozen" fight-or-flight response that can result from shock or emotional trauma.

The practitioner might talk during the massage to encourage the receiver to recognize any physical sensations that arise and to help them reconnect with their body. Involuntary reactions such as shivering, yawning, crying, sweating, and stomach noises indicate the release of tension and stress from unresolved and unexpressed emotions. The aim is for the body to "digest" and release stress, tension, and suppressed emotions, restoring energy flow and leaving a feeling of well-being, optimism, and balance.

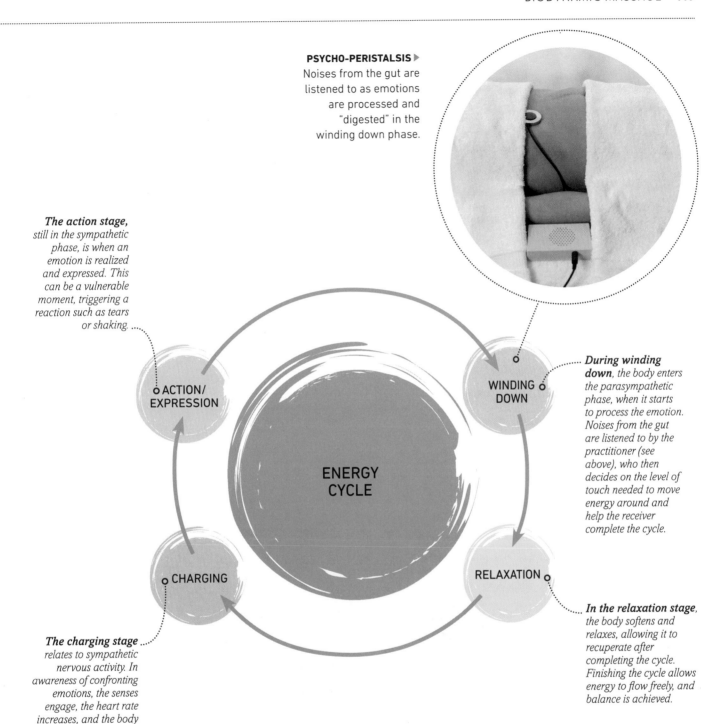

PSYCHO-PERISTALSIS ▶
Noises from the gut are listened to as emotions are processed and "digested" in the winding down phase.

The action stage, *still in the sympathetic phase, is when an emotion is realized and expressed. This can be a vulnerable moment, triggering a reaction such as tears or shaking.*

During winding down, the body enters the parasympathetic phase, when it starts to process the emotion. Noises from the gut are listened to by the practitioner (see above), who then decides on the level of touch needed to move energy around and help the receiver complete the cycle.

ACTION/ EXPRESSION

WINDING DOWN

ENERGY CYCLE

CHARGING

RELAXATION

The charging stage *relates to sympathetic nervous activity. In awareness of confronting emotions, the senses engage, the heart rate increases, and the body contracts, slowing down processes such as peristalsis in the gut. Energy moves from the core to the periphery to find expression.*

In the relaxation stage, *the body softens and relaxes, allowing it to recuperate after completing the cycle. Finishing the cycle allows energy to flow freely, and balance is achieved.*

▲ THE ENERGY CYCLE
The diagram above shows the energy cycle that biodynamic therapy works with. The four stages relate to activity in the parasympathetic and sympathetic nervous systems (see p.20). Energy can get stuck at any point, so the body doesn't recuperate and holds tension. During biodynamic massage, the practitioner helps the receiver complete the energy cycle to achieve balance and a healthy emotional state.

BIODYNAMIC MASSAGE

During biodynamic massage, the practitioner uses an electronic stethoscope to listen to the sounds of the gut, a practice known as psycho-peristalsis. Gurgling noises are positive, indicating that trapped emotions are being released and energy is flowing. Massage strokes are used, referred to as basic touch techniques in biodynamic practice, and work may also be done on the aura, or energy field.

BASIC TECHNIQUES USED
○ **Effleurage strokes, p.40**

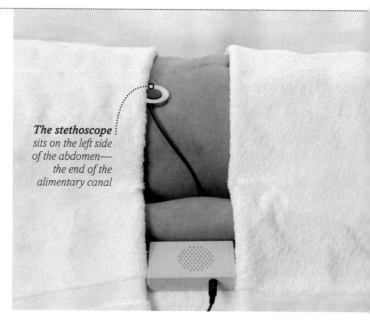

The stethoscope sits on the left side of the abdomen— the end of the alimentary canal

LISTENING TO THE GUT

▲ **At the start of the session**, an electronic stethoscope is placed on the abdomen. This is kept on the body throughout to listen to the gut and analyze whether emotions are blocked or released.

"EXITING" TECHNIQUE

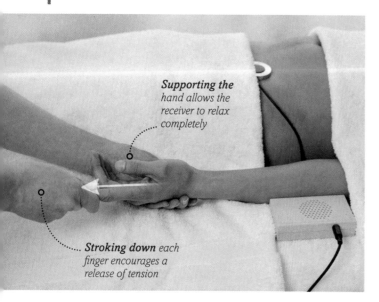

Supporting the hand allows the receiver to relax completely

Stroking down each finger encourages a release of tension

▲ **The "exiting" technique** involves stroking on the hands, feet, and head. Basic touch is used to relax the area while listening to the gut and observing breathing until a release of tension is sensed.

PALMING

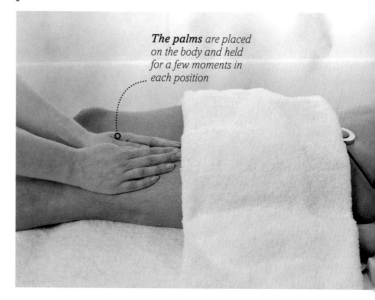

The palms are placed on the body and held for a few moments in each position

▲ **Palming is done** to contain and bring down energy. The whole body is worked on, traveling methodically from the head downward in a steady rhythm to create a sense of stability and calm.

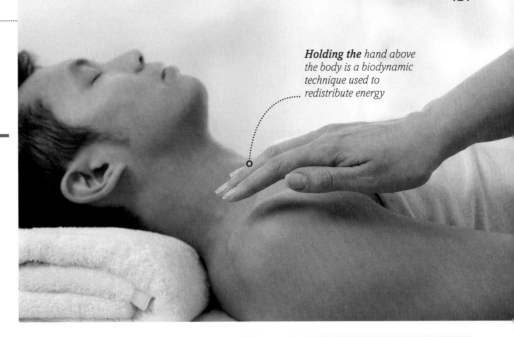

Holding the hand above the body is a biodynamic technique used to redistribute energy

WORKING ON THE AURA —

Biodynamic massage can ▶ involve working on the aura—or energy field—around the body to balance energy. This follows the principle that energy is released as we relax. This specialized technique can be beneficial if a person is frail or doesn't wish to be touched, guiding them to the spiritual side of their nature.

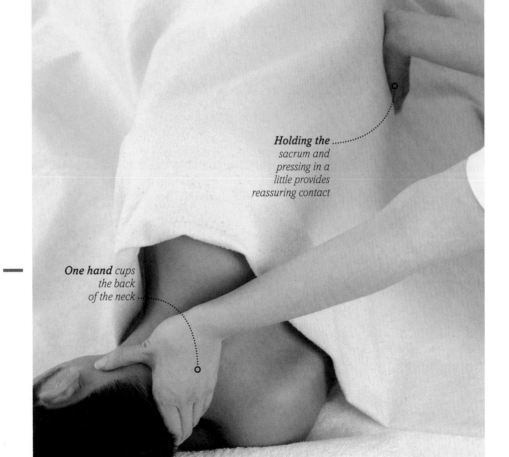

Holding the sacrum and pressing in a little provides reassuring contact

One hand cups the back of the neck

POLARIZATION —

This holding technique is done ▶ to close a session. The receiver lies on their left side, knees drawn up in the fetal position, and is covered with a blanket while the practitioner holds the neck and sacrum. Alternatively, a hold can be done on the abdomen or on the knees and ankles. This grounding, calming action can be held a little longer if agitated emotions need to be soothed.

KEY FACTS

ESSENCE	TECHNIQUES	BENEFITS
Smooth, heated stones are lightly oiled and used to massage and transfer heat.	Stones are used as a massage tool in adapted effleurage techniques.	Heat eases pain, reduces muscle tension, and increases tissue pliability.

SPECIALTIES

HOT STONE MASSAGE

There is a long history of using stones in healing and massage. In China, India, North and South America, Africa, Europe, and Egypt, the traditional use of stones includes practices such as placing them in patterns on the body, wearing stones to help improve health, or using stones in the treatment of pain and illness. The use of heated stones to improve the health of internal organs was documented more than 2,000 years ago in China. Today's hot stone massage derives from a practice called LaStone Therapy, started in 1993 by Mary Nelson, a massage therapist from Arizona.

HOW DOES HOT STONE MASSAGE WORK?

Nelson, the pioneer of hot stone massage therapy, felt spiritually guided to the healing properties of stones and heat and their combined ability to open energy channels. Today's practice builds on her principles, using heated stones as tools to relax and to soothe chronic pain. Hot stone massage adapts techniques from a variety of disciplines, including Swedish, deep tissue therapy, meridian therapy, and trigger point therapy.

In a hot stone massage, different-sized smooth stones (usually basalt) are heated in a water bath to around 126°F (52°C), then oil is applied to them instead of to the hands so the stones can move smoothly over the skin. Large stones may be placed on points on the body over a towel or sheet or on their own once the stone has transferred some of its heat in the massage. It is very important for the massage therapist to take care when leaving stones in one place on the body. He or she needs to ensure that the stones are sufficiently cooled so there is no chance of them burning the skin.

The heat from the stones boosts blood supply to an area; reduces muscle contraction; encourages relaxation; and helps relieve tense, painful muscles. Using stones also allows the practitioner to work into deeper muscle layers without straining the fingers, while the heat increases the pliability of muscles and connective tissue, making it easier to work into the tissues. Pressure can be adapted by using different parts of the stone; for example, deeper pressure can be applied with the edge of a stone.

STONE SIZES AND USES

The chart shows a non-life-size representation of different-sized stones and how these might be used. Great care needs to be taken to ensure that stones are the right temperature and that they are not left in one place for too long (see opposite).

WHERE THE STONE IS USED	TYPE OF STONE	HOW THE STONE IS USED
Mainly on larger areas, such as the back and the upper legs, and sometimes on the abdomen.	*Large, flat oval-shaped stone*	Large stones hold heat for longer, so they are suitable for making slow, deep strokes over large areas such as the back. They can be left on the lower back to keep this warm while smaller stones massage the back and legs.
These are commonly used on the back, upper legs, arms, and abdomen.	*Medium, flat oval-shaped stone*	These are useful for working over the shoulders and up into the neck. They are also a good size for the receiver to hold on the abdomen to keep this area warm while the upper body is massaged.
These smaller stones are ideal for working over the feet, hands, arms, legs, and into the neck.	*Small, flat oval-shaped stone*	Smaller stones retain heat for less time, so strokes tend to be faster and lighter. They are also easier to handle and manipulate, so they are ideal for negotiating smaller parts of the body.
Used mainly on the face and on small areas, such as the hands and feet.	*Extra small, flat oval-shaped stone*	These can be used to make small, gentle rotations over the face and head, avoiding the area around the eyes.
These can be placed and held between the toes and may also be used over the hands, feet, and head.	*Small round stones*	These stones fit perfectly in between the toes, so they can be left in place while small stones work on other parts of the feet and the lower legs.

HOT STONE MASSAGE

A hot stone massage session begins with a consultation where the practitioner checks whether there are any particular concerns. Usually a whole-body massage is carried out with the preheated stones, covering them in a little oil so they glide over the skin in smooth effleurage strokes. When they have transferred some of their heat, they can be safely left briefly in one place to warm the area. The heat, healing stones, and oils create an intensely relaxing experience. Here are some of the ways in which stones are used.

BASIC TECHNIQUES USED
○ **Slide and glide, p.44**
○ **Fan stroke, p.40**

USING LARGE STONES

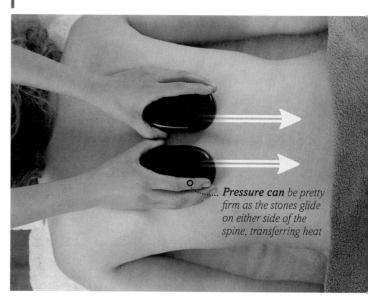

Pressure can be pretty firm as the stones glide on either side of the spine, transferring heat

▲ **Large stones** hold heat longer, so they are useful on big areas such as the back and thighs, where they can be used in sweeping effleurage strokes to warm up the tissues at the start of a back massage.

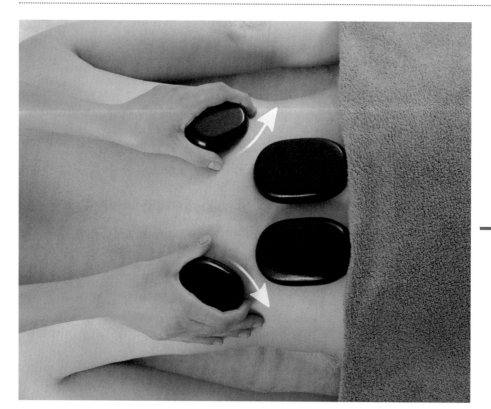

— HOLDING IN HEAT

◀ **Stones can** be left briefly in one place to transfer heat. Here, the larger stones that started the massage have transferred some of their heat and can be left safely to warm the muscular lower back area while medium-sized stones continue massaging over the back and/or the legs. The larger stones are then removed.

WORKING ON THE FEET ___

Small stones can be placed ▶ between the toes, which are often scrunched, tense, and cold. The stones will stay in place naturally between the toes, giving the feet a nice melting sensation, while larger stones are used to massage the feet and legs.

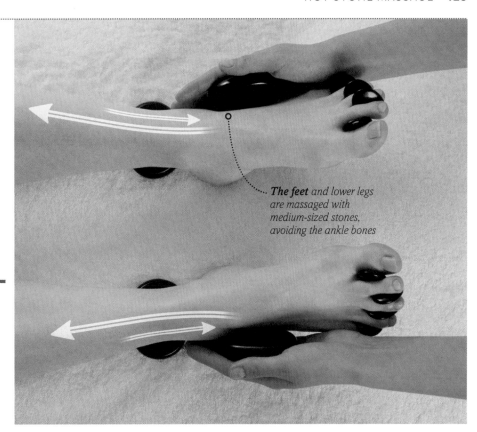

The feet and lower legs are massaged with medium-sized stones, avoiding the ankle bones

WARMING THE ABDOMEN

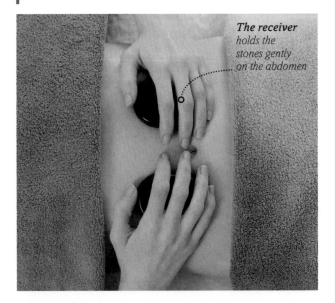

The receiver holds the stones gently on the abdomen

▲ **Toward the end** of a massage, the receiver can hold two stones on the abdomen. These act like a comforting hot water bottle while the practitioner works on the arms, upper chest, and head.

SMALL CIRCLES AND STATIC HOLDS

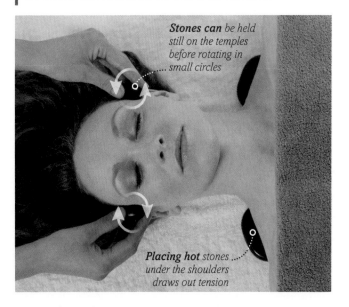

Stones can be held still on the temples before rotating in small circles

Placing hot stones under the shoulders draws out tension

▲ **A session ends** on the head and upper body, where small stones circle over the face, from jaw to temples. They can also be held under the nostrils, where heat can help clear the sinuses.

ESSENCE	TECHNIQUES	BENEFITS
Aids recovery from injuries or used as a pre- or postsporting event treatment.	Incorporates general massage styles and more specialized sports techniques.	Prevents injury, speeds recovery, and enhances athletic performance.

SPECIALTIES

SPORTS MASSAGE

One of the key roles of sports massage is to enhance the overall physical performance of a athlete both by warming up and softening tissues before an event—ensuring that muscles are working optimally—and also aiding recovery afterward to help flush out waste that accumulates with exercise and can harden tissues, causing stiffness. Integral to this work is the prevention of injury, and of course a therapist will help correct soft tissue damage when this does occur, whether through sports injuries or other injuries not directly related to sports.

HOW DOES SPORTS MASSAGE WORK?

A sports massage therapist has specific training for sports-related scenarios. A therapist may also suggest adjustments to training programs. For example, if a particularly tight muscle is observed, this can suggest the person isn't stretching the muscle sufficiently during training.

A variety of techniques is used during a sports massage session, including Swedish massage techniques such as effleurage and petrissage, deep tissue work, trigger point therapy, and assisted stretching.

In addition, a sports therapist may use specialized techniques such as muscle energy techniques (MET) (see opposite), which is where the receiver resists back against assisted stretches to help correct imbalances in muscle groups; myofascial release, where sustained pressure to an area releases tightness in the fascia; and neuromuscular techniques that address involuntary tension that is controlled by the nervous system. Acupuncture and acupressure may be used to work on pressure points around the body. A practitioner may also strap and tape certain muscles to help prevent injuries during training or an event and to treat existing injuries. The therapist may use a practice called gait analysis, as well as biodynamics, to study how someone holds themselves and moves to assess where problems may lie.

HAMSTRING CONTRACTING

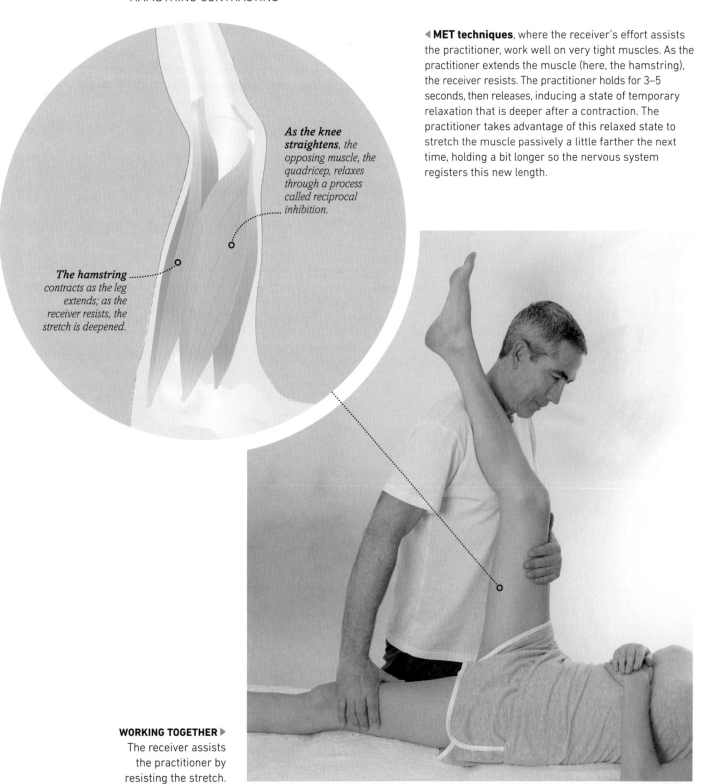

As the knee straightens, the opposing muscle, the quadricep, relaxes through a process called reciprocal inhibition.

The hamstring contracts as the leg extends; as the receiver resists, the stretch is deepened.

◄ **MET techniques**, where the receiver's effort assists the practitioner, work well on very tight muscles. As the practitioner extends the muscle (here, the hamstring), the receiver resists. The practitioner holds for 3–5 seconds, then releases, inducing a state of temporary relaxation that is deeper after a contraction. The practitioner takes advantage of this relaxed state to stretch the muscle passively a little farther the next time, holding a bit longer so the nervous system registers this new length.

WORKING TOGETHER ▶
The receiver assists the practitioner by resisting the stretch.

SPORTS MASSAGE

Sports massage is used to prevent injury, help muscles recover after an event, and treat injury. As well as effleurage, deep tissue work, and friction, trained practitioners use specialized techniques such as muscle energy techniques (MET) to test mobility and range of motion. With MET, the receiver resists a stretch applied by the practitioner. The pressure is released and then reapplied to help stretch muscles a little farther than they would usually go. Both receiver and practitioner use breaths to assist movements, exhaling into a stretch.

BASIC TECHNIQUES USED:
○ **Stretches, p.74**
○ **Effleurage, p.40**
○ **Petrissage, p.56**
○ **Passive movements, p.74**
○ **Pressure, p.72**
○ **Deep tissues massage, p.116**

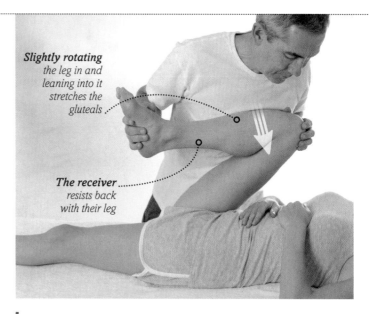

Slightly rotating the leg in and leaning into it stretches the gluteals

The receiver resists back with their leg

GLUTEAL STRETCH

▲ **The powerful gluteal muscles** help extend the hip and trunk and play a key role in sports, but overuse and repetitive actions can strain and tighten them. A gluteal stretch is a useful pre-event warm-up, usually done near the end of a session to stretch and release the warmed-up tissues.

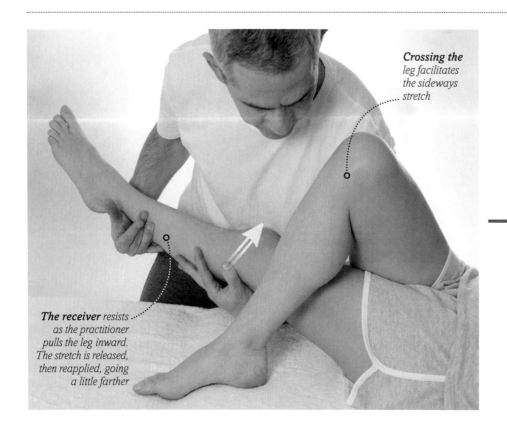

Crossing the leg facilitates the sideways stretch

The receiver resists as the practitioner pulls the leg inward. The stretch is released, then reapplied, going a little farther

STRETCHING THE IT BAND

◀ **The iliotibial (IT) band**, a tendon that runs from a muscle in the hip down to the tibia bone, helps stabilize the knee. It can tighten over time, mainly in runners, rubbing and causing inflammation. Combining a stretch to the IT band with MET techniques can help release tissue adhesions to reduce pain and increase mobility.

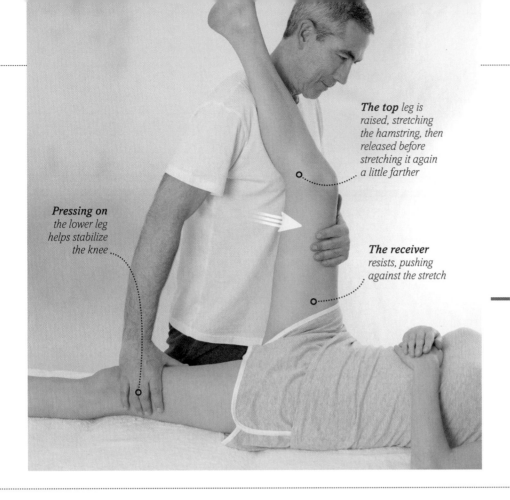

Pressing on the lower leg helps stabilize the knee

The top leg is raised, stretching the hamstring, then released before stretching it again a little farther

The receiver resists, pushing against the stretch

HAMSTRING STRETCH

◀ **The hamstrings** at the back of the thigh help stabilize the knee and the lower leg. Strains are common, and these muscles are often tight. As well as warm-up effleurage and deep tissue work, MET techniques can help release very tight hamstrings, helping muscles stretch slightly farther than they are used to doing.

FLEXING THE HIPS

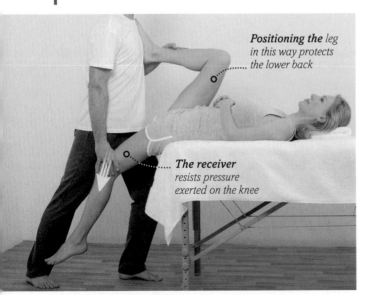

Positioning the leg in this way protects the lower back

The receiver resists pressure exerted on the knee

▲ **The hip flexor muscles**, which connect the legs and trunk, can become tight or strained. This move using MET techniques stretches these muscles to improve mobility and release lower back tension.

WHOLE-BODY STRETCH

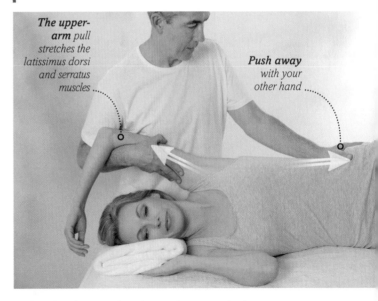

The upper-arm pull stretches the latissimus dorsi and serratus muscles

Push away with your other hand

▲ **This side-lying action** gives a nice upper-body stretch, relieving tightness in the hips, opening the chest, and releasing shoulder tension. The receiver exhales into the stretch to enhance the action.

ESSENCE	TECHNIQUES	BENEFITS
Painful nodules in a muscle refer pain. Treating this trigger eases the distant pain.	Manual treatment involves compression of the trigger point and stretching.	Using trigger point therapy helps treat and resolve chronic pain.

HOW DOES TRIGGER POINT THERAPY WORK?

By mapping out trigger point pathways throughout the body, Dr. Travell was able to find and treat the source of an individual's pain, even when this was distant from the area where the pain was actually felt. Massage therapists today approach their treatment in a more informed manner thanks to the pain patterns that she documented.

To locate a trigger point, the practitioner observes the receiver's pattern of pain, then probes the muscle that they suspect the pain originates from to establish its exact source. When the trigger point is compressed by the practitioner, the receiver feels a "good pain" and also experiences a reproduction of the pain pattern, which helps the practitioner confirm and treat the source of the pain.

Trigger points are treated in several ways. Massage therapists, physiotherapists, and osteopaths often use acupuncture as part of their practice or take a manual approach, using fingers, hands, or elbows to apply sustained compression to the trigger point, followed by a passive stretch to the area. Practitioners usually apply trigger point therapy during a general massage using Swedish and deep tissue techniques to soften and relax the tissues. Other trigger point treatments include the "spray and stretch" technique, favored by Dr. Travell, whereby a cooling spray anesthetizes the area before passively stretching it, or a corticosteroid injection can be given by a medical practitioner to relieve pain.

SPECIALTIES

TRIGGER POINT THERAPY

A trigger point is a nodule in a tight band of muscle that may cause local pain; a predictable pattern of referred pain; or autonomic symptoms such as tears, visual disturbances, and dizziness. Trigger point therapy was pioneered in the mid-20th century by a physician named Dr. Janet Travell—the personal physician to President Kennedy—who mapped patterns of referred pain associated with trigger points within specific muscles.

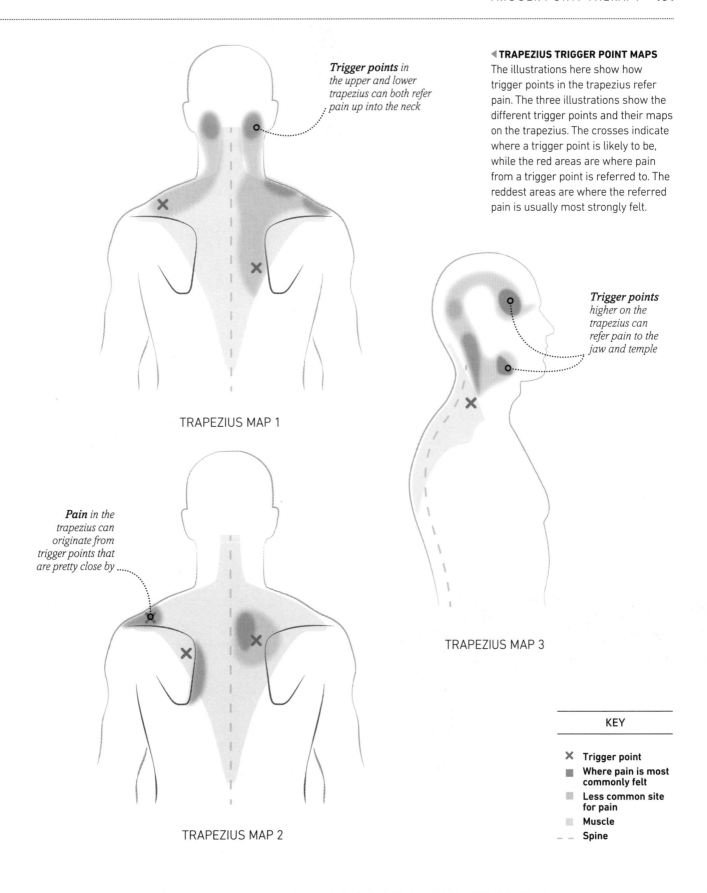

Trigger points in the upper and lower trapezius can both refer pain up into the neck

◄**TRAPEZIUS TRIGGER POINT MAPS**
The illustrations here show how trigger points in the trapezius refer pain. The three illustrations show the different trigger points and their maps on the trapezius. The crosses indicate where a trigger point is likely to be, while the red areas are where pain from a trigger point is referred to. The reddest areas are where the referred pain is usually most strongly felt.

TRAPEZIUS MAP 1

Trigger points higher on the trapezius can refer pain to the jaw and temple

Pain in the trapezius can originate from trigger points that are pretty close by

TRAPEZIUS MAP 3

TRAPEZIUS MAP 2

KEY	
✕	Trigger point
▇	Where pain is most commonly felt
▇	Less common site for pain
▇	Muscle
– –	Spine

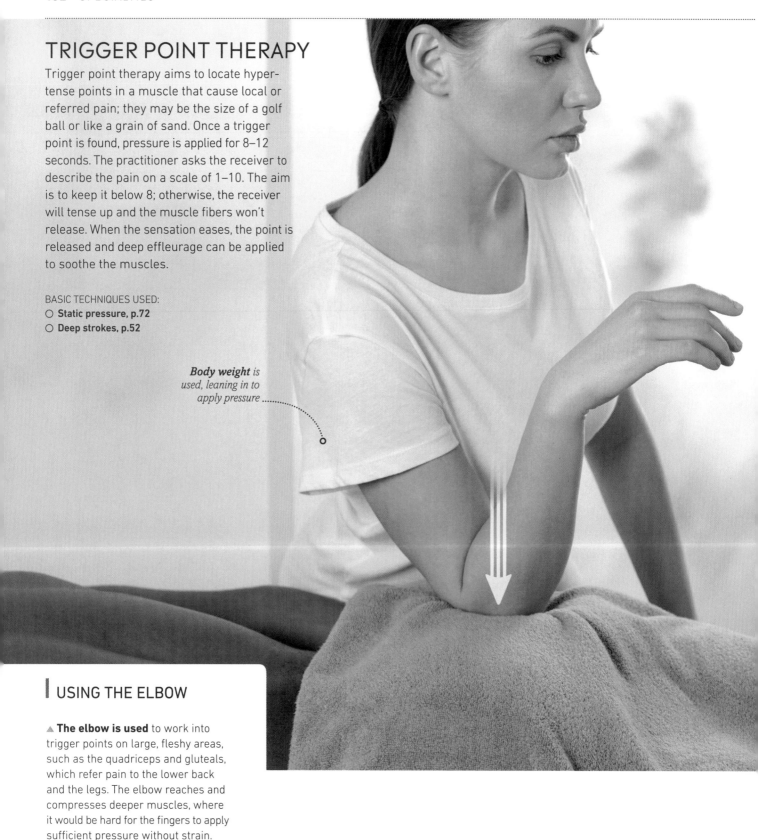

TRIGGER POINT THERAPY

Trigger point therapy aims to locate hyper-tense points in a muscle that cause local or referred pain; they may be the size of a golf ball or like a grain of sand. Once a trigger point is found, pressure is applied for 8–12 seconds. The practitioner asks the receiver to describe the pain on a scale of 1–10. The aim is to keep it below 8; otherwise, the receiver will tense up and the muscle fibers won't release. When the sensation eases, the point is released and deep effleurage can be applied to soothe the muscles.

BASIC TECHNIQUES USED:
○ **Static pressure, p.72**
○ **Deep strokes, p.52**

Body weight is used, leaning in to apply pressure

▌ USING THE ELBOW

▲ **The elbow is used** to work into trigger points on large, fleshy areas, such as the quadriceps and gluteals, which refer pain to the lower back and the legs. The elbow reaches and compresses deeper muscles, where it would be hard for the fingers to apply sufficient pressure without strain.

"The compression of a trigger point should be bearable; otherwise, the pressure is too deep."

"STRIPPING" THE MUSCLE

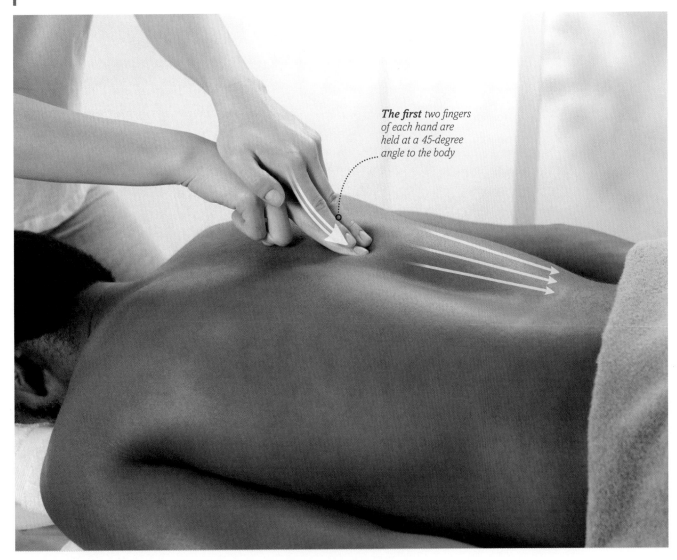

The first *two fingers of each hand are held at a 45-degree angle to the body*

▲ **This technique,** called "stripping the muscle," works on the erector spinae muscles on the back. The practitioner covers the whole muscle by working down three long strips in turn on either side of the spine. As the fingers slide down the erectors using deep pressure, the practitioner pauses where trigger points are detected.

SPECIALTIES

MANUAL LYMPHATIC DRAINAGE

Manual lymphatic drainage (MLD) is a type of massage that is used to help drain excess fluid from body tissues where this has accumulated and caused swelling. The practice was pioneered in the 1930s by Emil and Estrid Vodder after many years of research into the lymphatic system; all other types of MLD, including the Földi and Casley-Smith techniques, derive from the Vodder school. Emil and Estrid Vodder devised a system of light pumping movements to increase the absorption of excess fluids while avoiding blood becoming congested in one area.

KEY FACTS

ESSENCE	TECHNIQUES	BENEFITS
MLD manipulates the flow of lymph fluid through the lymphatic system.	A very light pumping action is made on the skin rather than deep in the muscles.	Reduces swelling caused by the accumulation of excess fluid in an area of the body.

HOW DOES MLD WORK?

MLD is unique in the world of massage because of the light touch employed and the different focus, which aims to stimulate the lymph vessels close to the surface of the skin rather than the muscle tissues. The techniques are used to treat a range of conditions, in particular lymphedema. Usually, fluid is transported through the body via the lymphatic system and lymph nodes and back into the blood. With lymphedema, the circulation of fluid is interrupted or blocked due to factors such as immobility, surgery, or cancer treatment, causing an area of swelling as fluid accumulates between the cells rather than draining away.

The Vodder school of MLD uses a very light pumping action on the tissues, carried out without any oil directly on the skin—so avoiding working into the muscles, which stimulates the circulation and actually increases the production of lymph. The aim is to increase the contractions of the lymph vessels and, in turn, increase the absorption of excess lymphatic fluid into the lymph nodes so that this can be drained out of the body. The practitioner works on an unaffected area first to clear fluids here and create space in the vessels so that the excess fluid from the affected area has somewhere to move to as it is absorbed and travels through the lymphatic system. As well as helping drain excess fluid, MLD is also used to reduce pain and aid relaxation.

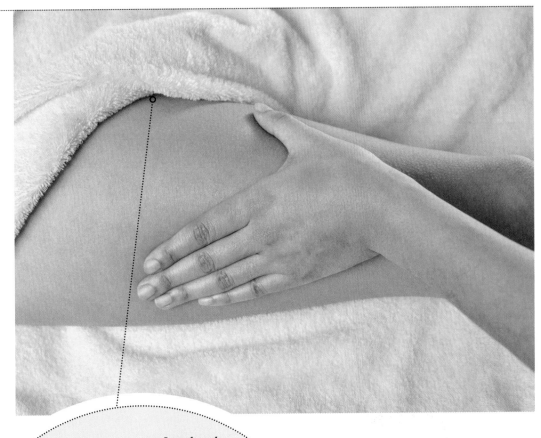

PUMP TECHNIQUE ▶
This pump action (see p.137) moves lymph fluid up into lymph nodes in the groin, where it is filtered and excess fluid drained.

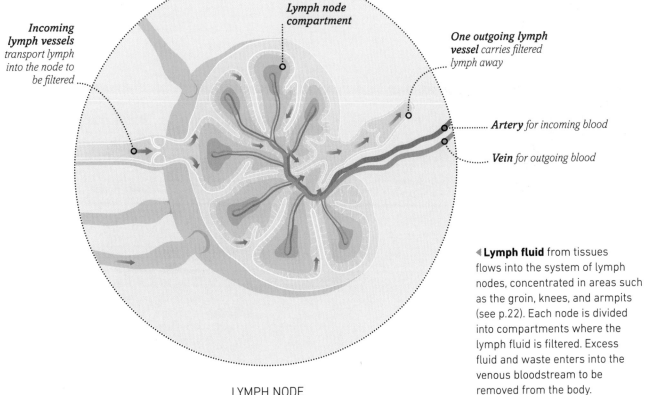

Incoming lymph vessels transport lymph into the node to be filtered

Lymph node compartment

One outgoing lymph vessel carries filtered lymph away

Artery for incoming blood

Vein for outgoing blood

LYMPH NODE

◀ **Lymph fluid** from tissues flows into the system of lymph nodes, concentrated in areas such as the groin, knees, and armpits (see p.22). Each node is divided into compartments where the lymph fluid is filtered. Excess fluid and waste enters into the venous bloodstream to be removed from the body.

MANUAL LYMPHATIC DRAINAGE (MLD)

NO BASIC TECHNIQUES USED:
In MLD, the focus is on stimulating lymph vessels close to the skin, not deeper muscle layers.

MLD uses very precise and light movements to move lymph through the lymph vessels to drain waste. No oil is used and the idea is that just the skin, not the muscle, is moved. The Vodder techniques shown below are basic treatments for common complaints such as headaches and fluid retention. More advanced techniques to treat conditions such as lymphedema require further training.

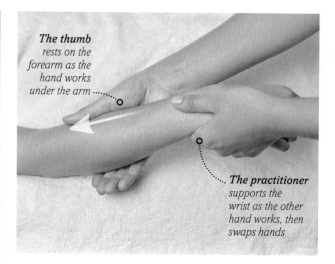

The thumb rests on the forearm as the hand works under the arm

The practitioner supports the wrist as the other hand works, then swaps hands

SCOOP

▲ **A scoop action** on the lower limbs follows the circling action, continuing to stimulate lymph up to the lymph nodes. The hands alternate in a light stretching (not sliding), pushing, and release action, moving up the arm to finish at the elbow.

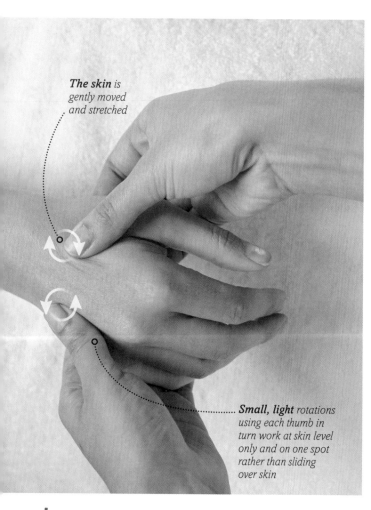

The skin is gently moved and stretched

Small, light rotations using each thumb in turn work at skin level only and on one spot rather than sliding over skin

THUMB CIRCLES

▲ **Light thumb circles** are used on small areas such as the wrist, feet, ankles, and hands. The subtle stretching and releasing action, repeated in a line over a hand or foot, is the start of a process to move lymph up to the auxiliary lymph nodes.

BEST HEIGHT
Light-touch MLD techniques require the massage table to be set pretty high, unlike other massages, where the practitioner lowers the table to lean in with their body weight.

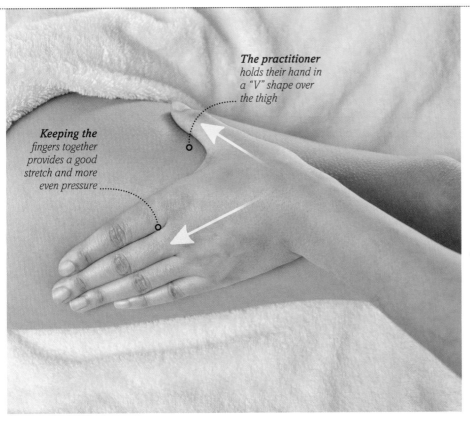

The practitioner holds their hand in a "V" shape over the thigh

Keeping the fingers together provides a good stretch and more even pressure

— PUMP

◀ **This stretch and release** action is suitable on the upper limbs—in particular, the thigh, where there is a larger surface area. As with the scoop, the aim is to stretch the skin only, then release, repeating this action as you work up the limb to encourage excess fluid into the lymph nodes.

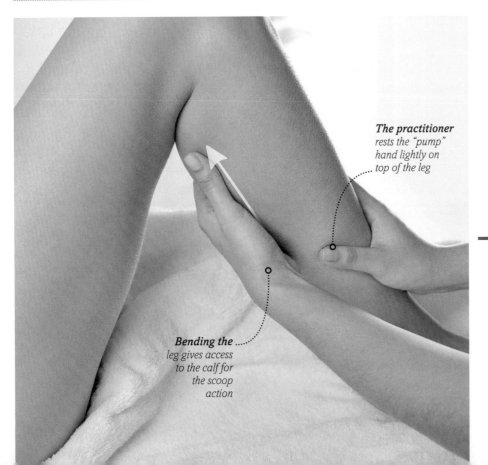

The practitioner rests the "pump" hand lightly on top of the leg

Bending the leg gives access to the calf for the scoop action

— PUMP SCOOP

◀ **This action**, done on the calf, combines the techniques of the pump and scoop to maximize lymph drainage. The pump and release action is done with the top hand, followed by the scoop and release action with the bottom hand, working up the limb to finish before the knee.

KEY FACTS

ESSENCE	TECHNIQUES	BENEFITS
Ayurvedic massage is part of the wider field of Ayurvedic medicine.	Treats via the senses with massage, infused oils, music, and visualizations.	Maintains energy balance in the body and erases physical tensions caused by stress.

SPECIALTIES

AYURVEDIC MASSAGE

Ayurveda means "the science of life" in Sanskrit and stems from the ancient Vedic culture, which originated over 5,000 years ago in India. Ayurvedic massage is a key part of Ayurvedic medicine and the Ayurvedic way of life, a truly holistic system that embraces yoga, nutrition, herbal medicine, cleansing rituals called panchakarma, and meditation. In Ayurvedic tradition, everything in the universe is made up of five elements that join in the body to create three types of energy, or doshas, called Vata, Pitta, and Kapha. Ayurveda aims to keep these doshas in balance because when there is minimal stress and energy flow is balanced, the body is well-equipped to defend itself from disease.

HOW DOES AYURVEDIC MASSAGE WORK?

Ayurvedic massage is one of the tools that is used in Ayurvedic practice to help rebalance energy; revitalize and relax the body; and strengthen body, mind, and spirit.

At an initial consultation, the practitioner observes the different layers of the person's pulse, listens to the tone of their voice, examines their tongue and eyes, and observes their general physique. These various observations help the practitioner to determine the herbs, base oils, essential oils, music (known as ragas), mantras, and guided visualizations (known as sankalpas) that will be used during the massage treatment.

The selected herbs are steeped in oil, which is warmed before the massage. During the massage, generous quantities of this herb-infused oil are used to help open and cleanse the energy channels in the body. The practitioner uses a combination of lighter and deeper strokes, although the amount of oil means that strokes are generally lighter than other types of massage, with the focus more on the gliding action than on working deep into tissues. Long, gliding strokes follow the energy channels of the body and work on the nerves, and pinching or kneading are also used to help release tension caused by the unconscious guarding of the body in response to emotional stress.

Marma points—points found on the energy channels (see opposite)—and the chakras (see p.165) are treated to assist the flow of vital energy, and the whole body is massaged, giving a feeling of integration and full-body awareness.

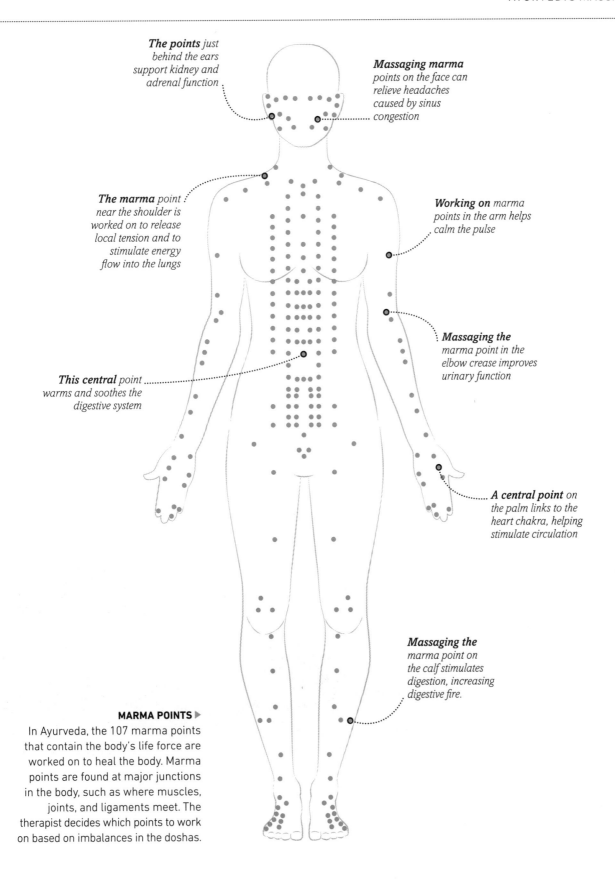

The points *just behind the ears support kidney and adrenal function*

Massaging marma *points on the face can relieve headaches caused by sinus congestion*

The marma *point near the shoulder is worked on to release local tension and to stimulate energy flow into the lungs*

Working on *marma points in the arm helps calm the pulse*

Massaging the *marma point in the elbow crease improves urinary function*

This central *point warms and soothes the digestive system*

A central point *on the palm links to the heart chakra, helping stimulate circulation*

Massaging the *marma point on the calf stimulates digestion, increasing digestive fire.*

MARMA POINTS ▶

In Ayurveda, the 107 marma points that contain the body's life force are worked on to heal the body. Marma points are found at major junctions in the body, such as where muscles, joints, and ligaments meet. The therapist decides which points to work on based on imbalances in the doshas.

AYURVEDIC MASSAGE

Ayurvedic massage is just one aspect of Ayurvedic holistic healing and can be enjoyed on its own or as part of a complete Ayurvedic way of life to balance the body's energy. Long, sweeping, quick movements are typical, using plenty of oil to facilitate a light, gliding action. The practitioner's training allows them to tailor the massage to focus on marma points and balancing the doshas (see p.138).

BASIC TECHNIQUES USED:
O **Slide and glide, p.44**

| WORKING AROUND MARMA POINTS

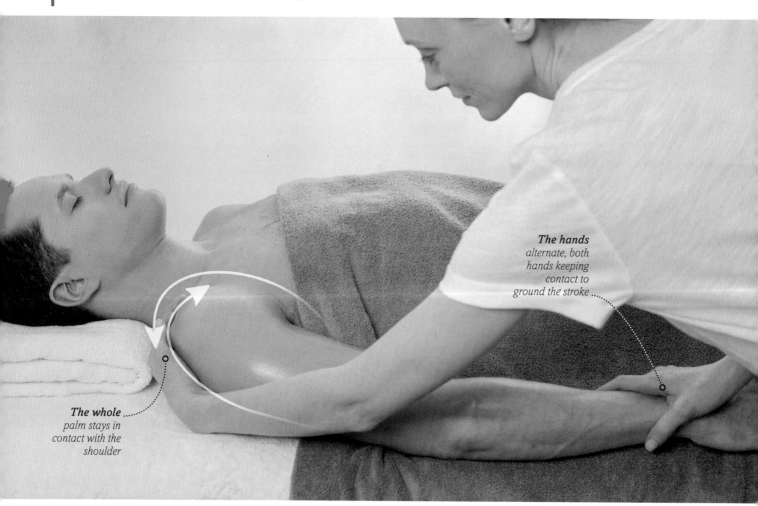

The hands alternate, both hands keeping contact to ground the stroke

The whole palm stays in contact with the shoulder

▲ **Working into the marma point** at the top of the shoulder helps release blocked energy here, releasing local tension, as well as stress around the body. After effleuraging the arm with fast, long strokes, the practitioner works extensively on the shoulder, circling clockwise and counterclockwise.

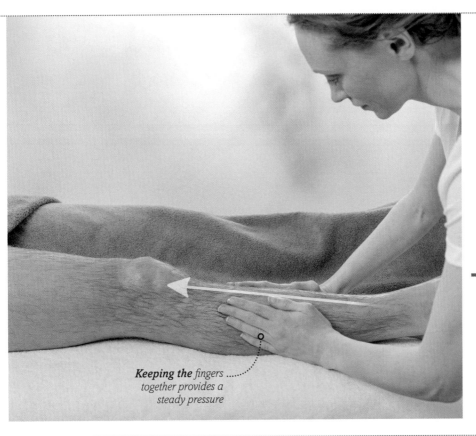

Keeping the fingers
*together provides a
steady pressure*

STROKES TO CALM EXCESS ENERGY

◀ **Long, gliding, rhythmic** strokes that travel up the whole leg are used to help calm excess energy, or fire, to bring balance to the body. With the hands on the sides of the leg, the practitioner lunges in to glide up the whole limb, using one long sweeping action.

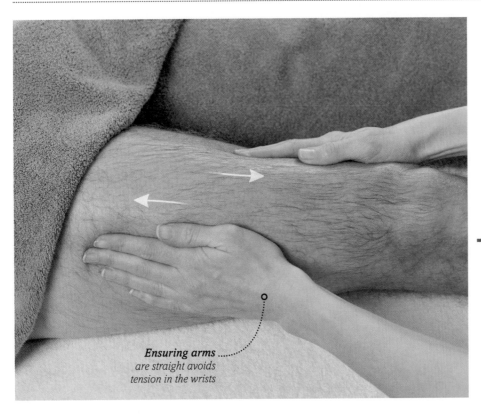

*Ensuring arms
are straight avoids
tension in the wrists*

ENERGIZING TECHNIQUES

◀ **Lively strokes to the legs** may be prescribed to reenergize and invigorate the body when there is sluggishness and a lack of energy. Here, short rubbing strokes are applied to the fleshy thigh, alternating the hands back and forth to stimulate the tissues and energize the whole body.

HOW DOES THAI MASSAGE WORK?

During Thai massage, the practitioner uses a range of techniques and "body work" to remove restrictions to the flow of energy throughout the body to achieve balance and harmony and optimize health.

A Thai massage treatment is carried out on the floor on a mat or a mattress, with both the practitioner and receiver dressed in loose-fitting, comfortable clothing that doesn't restrict movements. The practitioner presses on points on Sen channels—using their feet, palms, thumbs, elbows, or knees—applying deep, careful pressure with these different parts of the body to remove blockages and encourage energy flow. Strong stretches and twists are also used to improve flexibility and muscle tone, which in turn helps reduce muscular pain. This body work is sometimes described as applied or assisted yoga as the practitioner moves themselves and the receiver into different positions in a fluid, unhurried manner, assisting the receiver to help them achieve certain stretches without strain. The massage has the effect of increasing overall vitality and flexibility, reducing pain, and leaving the receiver with a feeling of deep relaxation.

Relevant training is needed to master the practice. Knowledge has been handed down from generation to generation in Thailand, leading to some differences in style and techniques between regions and also individual practitioners.

MASSAGE SPECIALTIES
THAI MASSAGE

Thai massage is one of the elements of traditional Thai medicine, believed in folklore to have been created by a friend and physician to the Buddha some 2,500 years ago. The massage was seen as a spiritual practice, done in Buddhist temples, and carvings documenting techniques can be seen at the Wat Pho temple complex in Thailand. Thai medicine is based on the principle that areas where energy stagnates or is depleted cause pain and disease. The aim of Thai massage is to optimize energy flow through channels in the body known as Sen (see opposite) to balance energy and promote healing and health in body and mind.

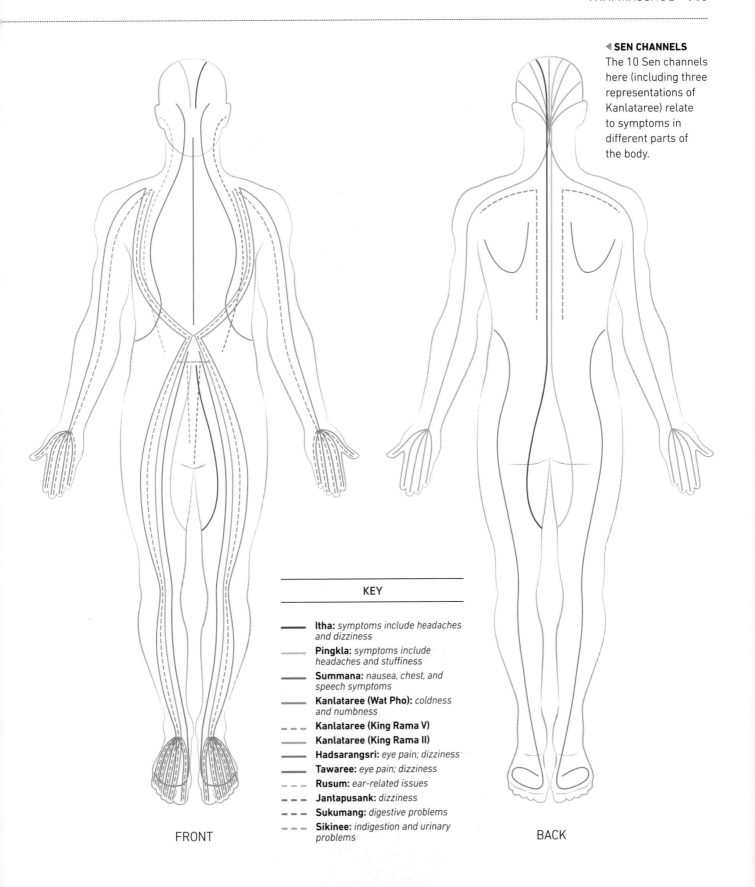

◀ **SEN CHANNELS**
The 10 Sen channels here (including three representations of Kanlataree) relate to symptoms in different parts of the body.

KEY

— **Itha:** *symptoms include headaches and dizziness*

— **Pingkla:** *symptoms include headaches and stuffiness*

— **Summana:** *nausea, chest, and speech symptoms*

— **Kanlataree (Wat Pho):** *coldness and numbness*

- - - **Kanlataree (King Rama V)**

— — **Kanlataree (King Rama II)**

— **Hadsarangsri:** *eye pain; dizziness*

— **Tawaree:** *eye pain; dizziness*

- - - **Rusum:** *ear-related issues*

- - - **Jantapusank:** *dizziness*

- - - **Sukumang:** *digestive problems*

- - - **Sikinee:** *indigestion and urinary problems*

FRONT

BACK

THAI MASSAGE

A Thai massage energizes the body by working on pressure points to release energy and carrying out assisted yoga stretches to release tension and increase flexibility. There is no need for the receiver to be flexible—the practitioner will use their expertise to take the client a little further than they would normally go, always being mindful of their limitations. All the techniques require relevant training.

BASIC TECHNIQUES USED
○ **Petrissage, p.56**
○ **Effleurage, p.40**
○ **Pressure, p.72**

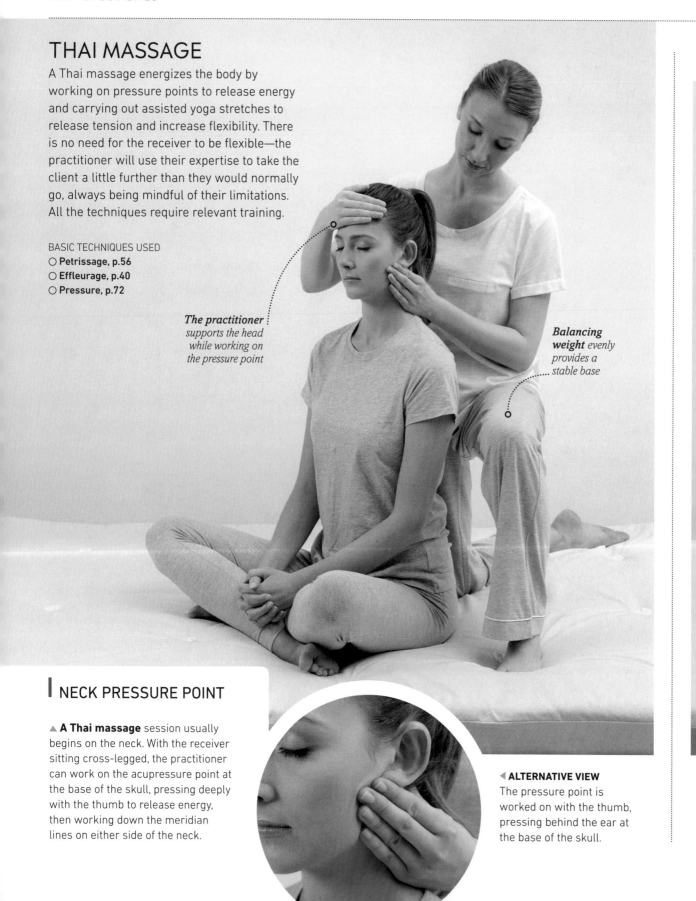

The practitioner supports the head while working on the pressure point

Balancing weight evenly provides a stable base

NECK PRESSURE POINT

▲ **A Thai massage** session usually begins on the neck. With the receiver sitting cross-legged, the practitioner can work on the acupressure point at the base of the skull, pressing deeply with the thumb to release energy, then working down the meridian lines on either side of the neck.

◀ **ALTERNATIVE VIEW**
The pressure point is worked on with the thumb, pressing behind the ear at the base of the skull.

FOREARM PRESSURE

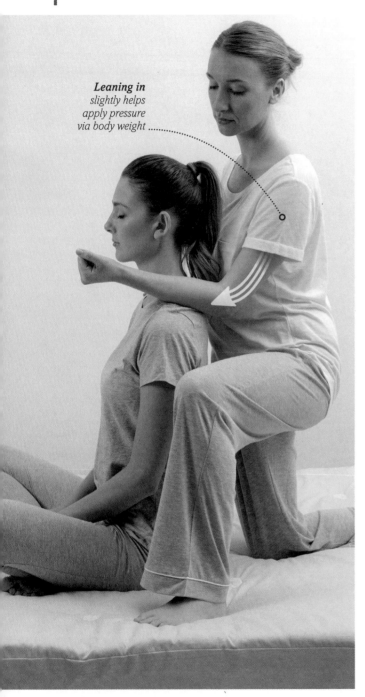

Leaning in slightly helps apply pressure via body weight

▲ **The shoulders** are also worked on while the receiver is seated. From a kneeling position, the practitioner's forearm can press down deeply on the trapezius, helping relax tissues and release tension.

SIDE-LYING LEG STRETCH

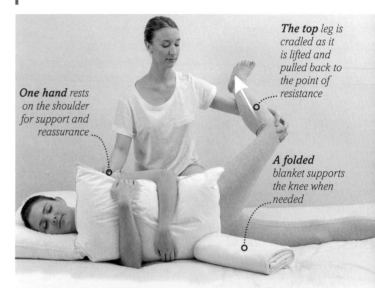

The top leg is cradled as it is lifted and pulled back to the point of resistance

One hand rests on the shoulder for support and reassurance

A folded blanket supports the knee when needed

▲ **Side-lying positions** facilitate work on the limbs. The receiver uses pillows for support and the practitioner presses into the hip with their knee to stabilize the body while stretching the limb.

FOOT PRESSURE

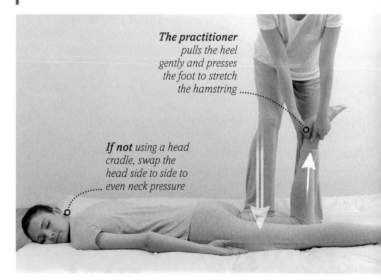

The practitioner pulls the heel gently and presses the foot to stretch the hamstring

If not using a head cradle, swap the head side to side to even neck pressure

▲ **The feet** become a massage tool in Thai practice and can be used all over the body. Here, from standing, the foot is placed firmly on the thigh, pressing on the tissues while also working on pressure points on the leg.

CONTINUED ▶

THAI MASSAGE *continued*

ASSISTED BACK BEND

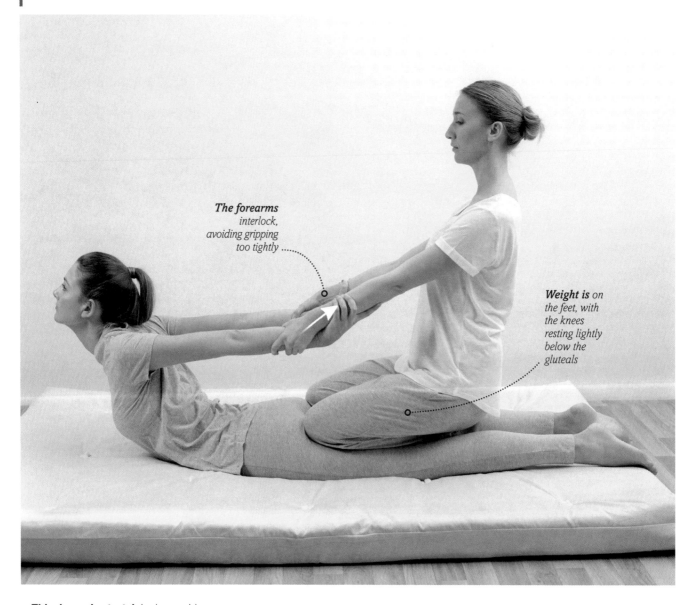

The forearms interlock, avoiding gripping too tightly .....

Weight is on the feet, with the knees resting lightly below the gluteals

▲ **This dynamic stretch** is done midmassage during back work. The practitioner asks the receiver to exhale while pulling them back, reminding the receiver to release their shoulders down, holding the position for 5 seconds.

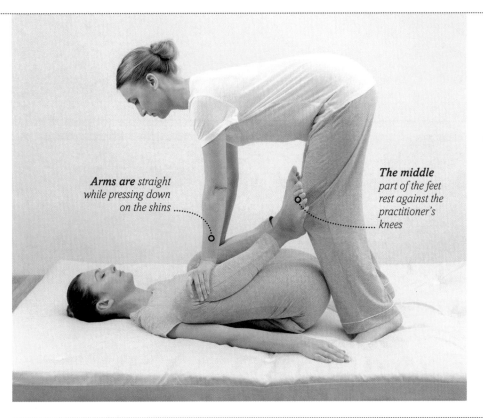

Arms are straight
while pressing down
on the shins ......

The middle
part of the feet
rest against the
practitioner's
knees

— BALL POSITION 1

◀ **This interactive** "ball" position
stretches the gluteus and lower
back muscles. The practitioner
pushes the lower legs firmly
into the ribcage until the point
of resistance is felt. Talk to and
observe the receiver to check
for tension. You can repeat the
move, guiding, with care, a little
past the point of resistance.

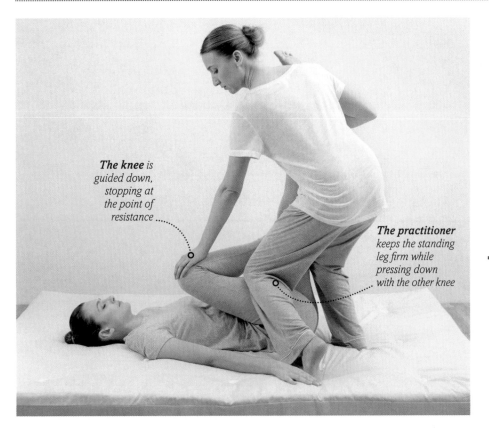

The knee is
guided down,
stopping at
the point of
resistance ......

The practitioner
keeps the standing
leg firm while
pressing down
with the other knee

— BALL POSITION 2

◀ **With the receiver** lying on
their back, one leg is pressed
in toward the chest and the
other leg held straight as the
practitioner puts firm pressure
on the hamstring with their
knee, stretching out the
muscles in the gluteals,
thighs, and the lower back.

CONTINUED ▶

THAI MASSAGE *continued*

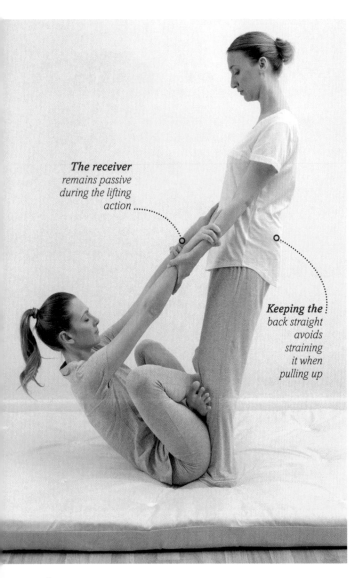

The receiver remains passive during the lifting action

Keeping the back straight avoids straining it when pulling up

PULLING UP

▲ **Pulling the receiver** up to sitting cross-legged from lying is an interactive way to change their position that also releases and straightens the back. Once the receiver is seated, the massage is brought to a close with assisted shoulder stretches and twists.

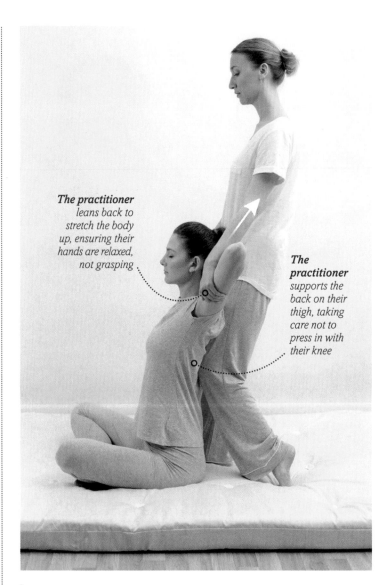

The practitioner leans back to stretch the body up, ensuring their hands are relaxed, not grasping

The practitioner supports the back on their thigh, taking care not to press in with their knee

CHEST OPENER

▲ **Assisted opening poses** are done toward the end of a session, opening up the chest area to give a nice sense of release. By positioning their thigh in the upper back, the practitioner can pull the receiver's body up into a gentle back bend, holding for 5 seconds.

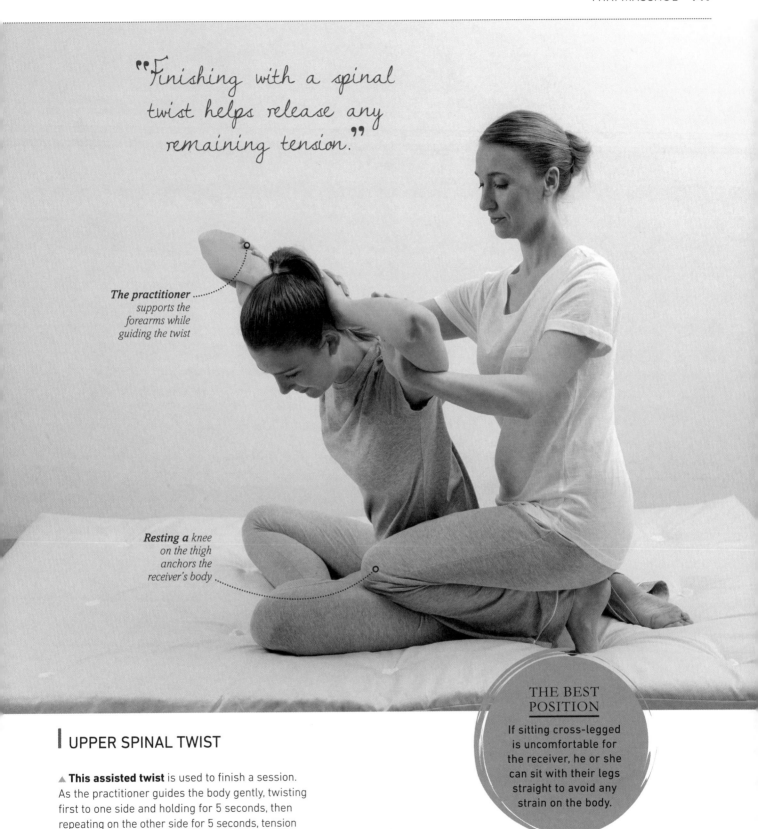

"Finishing with a spinal twist helps release any remaining tension."

The practitioner supports the forearms while guiding the twist

Resting a knee on the thigh anchors the receiver's body

UPPER SPINAL TWIST

▲ **This assisted twist** is used to finish a session. As the practitioner guides the body gently, twisting first to one side and holding for 5 seconds, then repeating on the other side for 5 seconds, tension is released in the upper back and shoulders.

THE BEST POSITION

If sitting cross-legged is uncomfortable for the receiver, he or she can sit with their legs straight to avoid any strain on the body.

KEY FACTS

ESSENCE	TECHNIQUES	BENEFITS
Principles of Chinese medicine are applied to diagnose energy flow in the body.	Manual techniques are used to restore balance to the flow of Qi.	Physical and emotional issues are improved once energy flow is restored.

MASSAGE SPECIALTIES

CHINESE TUI NA

Tui Na dates back over 3,000 years and is one of the four main branches of traditional Chinese medicine, which includes acupuncture, herbal medicine, and Qi Gong, a practice focused on posture and breathing. In Chinese medicine, all disease and disharmony is thought to be caused by an imbalance in the flow of energy, or Qi as it is referred to in China, which passes through the network of meridians in the body. Tui Na aims to treat the symptoms of specific illnesses, as well as address musculoskeletal complaints by restoring balance to the flow of energy throughout the body.

HOW DOES TUI NA WORK?

Tui Na massage is seen as a medical application of massage in China and has been continually refined by doctors in Chinese medical colleges and hospitals over its long history. Today, it continues to be very popular in China and is the first choice of treatment for infants and children, where techniques are suitably adapted. The practice is also beginning to gain popularity in the West.

In an initial consultation, the practitioner discusses topics such as sleep patterns, dietary habits, bowel movements, menstruation, and how a person is experiencing pain. The tongue, eyes, and skin are also examined, and the pulse is checked. Tui Na practitioners make a diagnosis based on the principles of energy flow in Chinese medicine before deciding on which approach to take in the massage.

Once a diagnosis is reached, the practitioner aims to resolve problems with energy flow by stimulating acupressure points (see opposite) along the meridians. A variety of techniques is used, including rapid repetitive movements with different parts of the hands and fingers, still compressions held for several minutes, and stretches and joint rotations. Treatments are usually carried out on a massage couch, either with the client dressed or with techniques applied to bare skin using a lubricant.

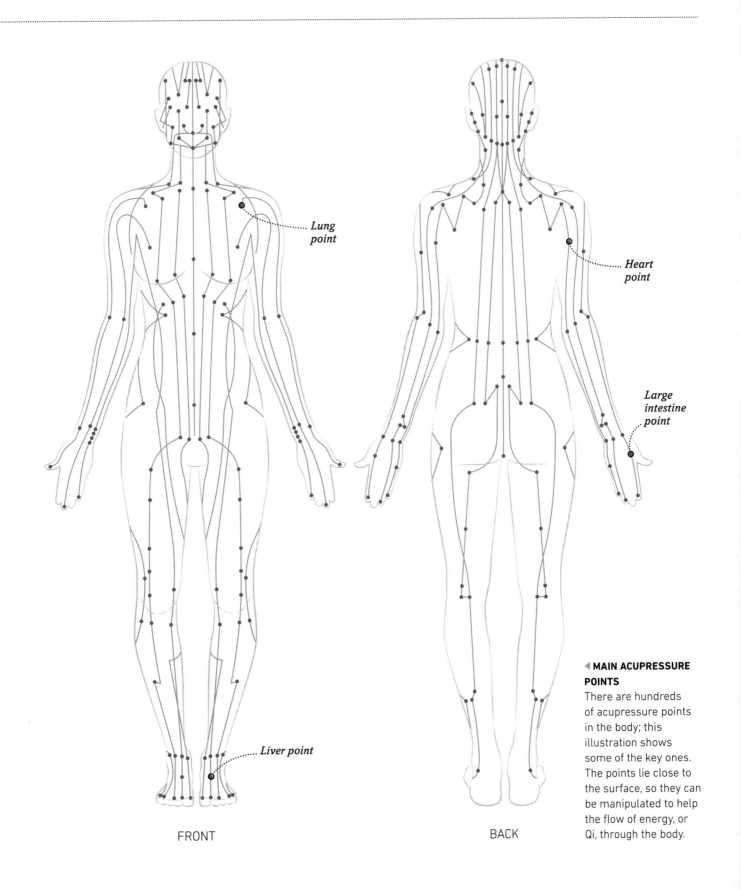

Lung point

Heart point

Large intestine point

Liver point

FRONT

BACK

◀ **MAIN ACUPRESSURE POINTS**
There are hundreds of acupressure points in the body; this illustration shows some of the key ones. The points lie close to the surface, so they can be manipulated to help the flow of energy, or Qi, through the body.

CHINESE TUI NA

After a consultation to talk about sleeping and eating patterns and a brief physical examination, the practitioner will make a diagnosis, deciding on where energy needs rebalancing in the body. As well as general, fairly fast effleurage, the practitioner may use techniques to stretch the tissues, as well as work on particular acupressure points to help unblock energy in parts of the body.

BASIC TECHNIQUES USED:
- Slide and glide, p.44
- Stretches, p.74
- Deep strokes, p.52
- Static pressure, p.72
- Knuckling, p.58

| STRETCHING THE TISSUES

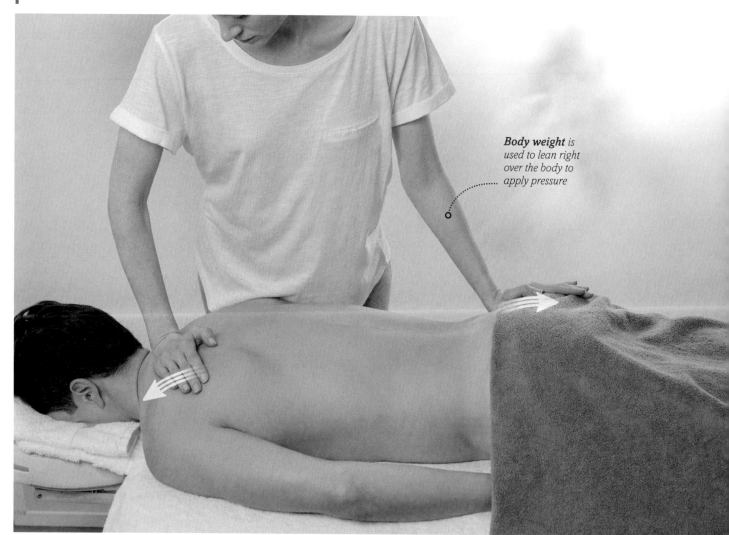

Body weight is used to lean right over the body to apply pressure

▲ **Stretching the whole back** warms tissues and releases the tension that can block energy flow. The practitioner presses into the fleshy shoulder and gluteal areas, stretching tissues out. This can also be done over a towel at the start of a treatment.

" The practitioner stimulates the points where energy needs rebalancing in the body."

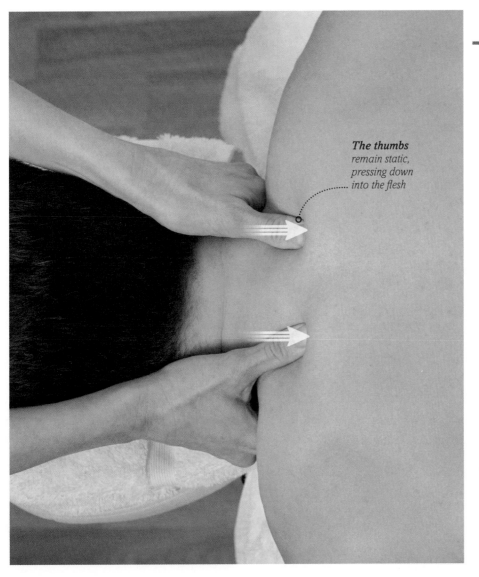

The thumbs remain static, pressing down into the flesh

WORKING ON PRESSURE POINTS

◀ **The thumbs** can be used to work into key acupressure points, releasing blockages to energy flow. The thumbs work deeply into the muscle to compress the tissues, holding them sometimes for several minutes. The knuckles can also be used to fan out over the upper trapezius once the pressure is released.

ADDITIONAL TREATMENTS

Some Tui Na practitioners are trained in (and insured for) moxibustion techniques—the burning of the herb mugwort—to enhance energy flow.

KEY FACTS

ESSENCE	TECHNIQUES	BENEFITS
Optimizes the flow of Ki through meridians to treat physical and emotional illness.	Still pressure is applied, together with stretching and rotation of limbs.	Promotes healing in the body and mind once blockages are released.

HOW DOES SHIATSU WORK?

There are many different styles of shiatsu that are practiced today. Some methods concentrate on particular acupressure points in the body; other practitioners focus more generally on the energy channels, called meridians (see opposite), to boost the flow of Ki throughout the body; while some practitioners focus on different traditional Chinese diagnostic systems.

However, all shiatsu practitioners diagnose and treat an individual according to the broad principles of traditional Chinese medicine, whereby malfunction and disease within the body and mind are believed to be caused by disruption to the flow of Ki through the meridians, or energy channels. Health concerns that disrupt the flow of blood and lymph in the body are also believed to affect the flow of Ki.

Shiatsu treatments are usually carried out on the floor with the practitioner and client dressed in loose-fitting, nonrestrictive clothing. The practitioner uses hand pressure and manipulative techniques to adjust the body's position to optimize the flow of Ki. Still, relaxed pressure is applied to various points on the body called tsubos, which lie along the meridian lines, and the assisted stretching and rotation of the person's limbs helps open up meridian lines to remove blockages.

MASSAGE SPECIALTIES

SHIATSU

Shiatsu is a Japanese word meaning "finger pressure." In shiatsu practice, pressure is applied to points on the body to help improve the flow of energy—or Ki in Japan—through the body to stimulate the body's natural healing powers. Shiatsu was developed in the early part of the 20th century by Japanese practitioner Tamai Tempaku. He incorporated medical knowledge of anatomy and physiology from the West into several older methods of traditional medicine, in particular drawing on an earlier form of Japanese massage called Anma, which in turn has its roots in traditional Chinese practices such as Tui Na (see p.150).

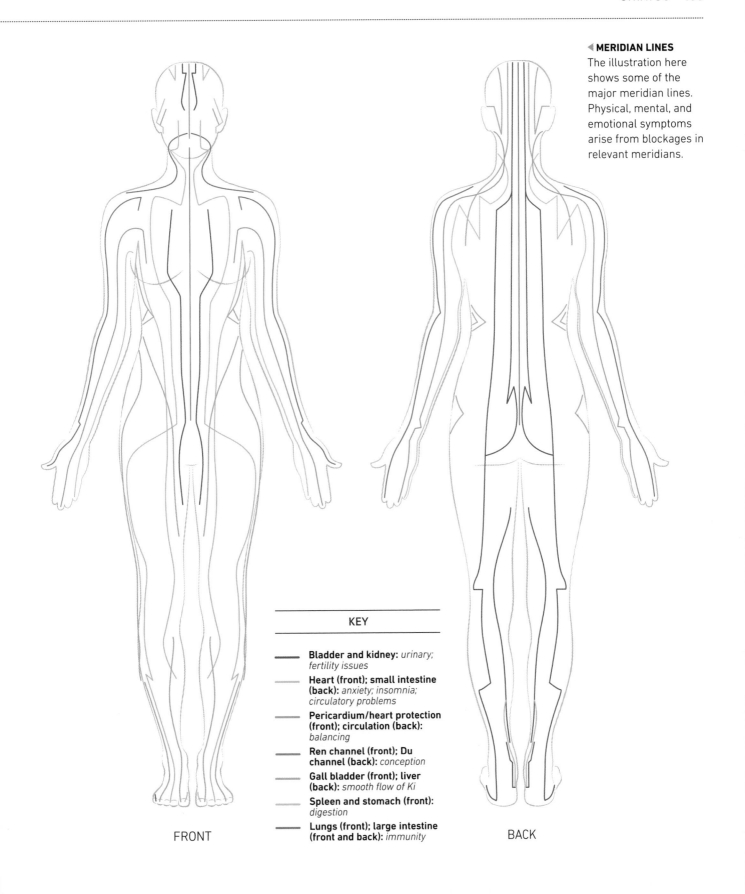

◀ **MERIDIAN LINES**
The illustration here shows some of the major meridian lines. Physical, mental, and emotional symptoms arise from blockages in relevant meridians.

KEY

— **Bladder and kidney:** *urinary; fertility issues*

— **Heart (front); small intestine (back):** *anxiety; insomnia; circulatory problems*

— **Pericardium/heart protection (front); circulation (back):** *balancing*

— **Ren channel (front); Du channel (back):** *conception*

— **Gall bladder (front); liver (back):** *smooth flow of Ki*

— **Spleen and stomach (front):** *digestion*

— **Lungs (front); large intestine (front and back):** *immunity*

FRONT

BACK

SHIATSU

Shiatsu is practiced on the floor with the client clothed. The practitioner is extremely calm and focused as he or she uses their own energy to balance and transmit energy—Ki—to the receiver. Still, relaxed pressure is applied at various points, called tsubos, on the meridian lines—with the quality of touch being more important than the pressure used—and stretching and rotating movements are done.

BASIC TECHNIQUES USED
○ **Static pressure, p.72**
○ **Passive movements, p.74**

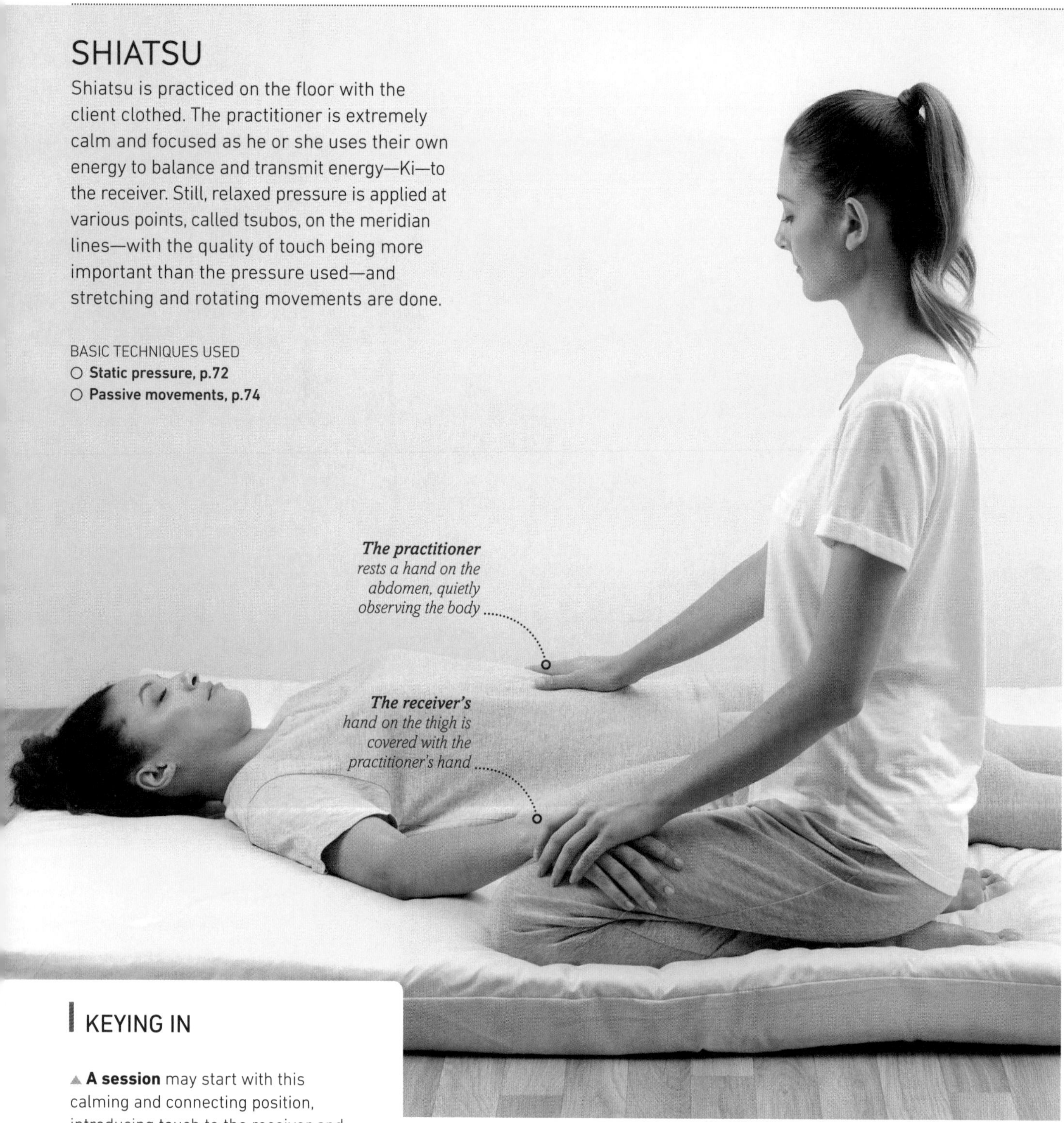

The practitioner
rests a hand on the
abdomen, quietly
observing the body

The receiver's
hand on the thigh is
covered with the
practitioner's hand

KEYING IN

▲ **A session** may start with this calming and connecting position, introducing touch to the receiver and building trust as the session begins. The practitioner creates a physical circle with the receiver, through contact and holding the receiver's hand, starting the dialogue of touch.

HARA DIAGNOSIS

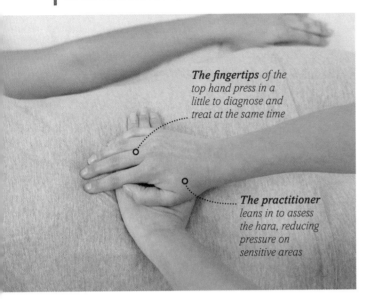

The fingertips of the top hand press in a little to diagnose and treat at the same time

The practitioner leans in to assess the hara, reducing pressure on sensitive areas

▲ **Palpating** the "hara" region on the abdomen—the vitality center of the body—helps to make a diagnosis. Tightness, warmth, tenderness, and sounds can all indicate areas that need attention.

PRESSURE POINT WORK

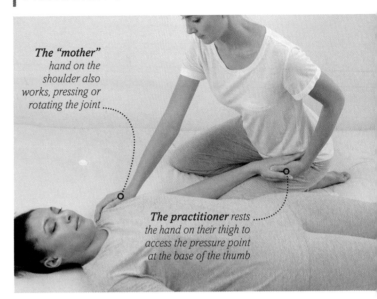

The "mother" hand on the shoulder also works, pressing or rotating the joint

The practitioner rests the hand on their thigh to access the pressure point at the base of the thumb

▲ **Working on pressure points** along meridian lines helps restore energy flow. The thumb pressure point is an important one, as it links to digestion and helps release pain.

WORKING AROUND THE HEAD

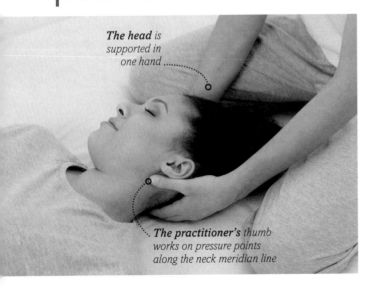

The head is supported in one hand

The practitioner's thumb works on pressure points along the neck meridian line

▲ **The head and neck** are worked on a great deal in shiatsu, as this area holds a lot of tension. The palms or the thumbs are used to work on pressure points in meridians over the head and neck.

USING THE FOREARM

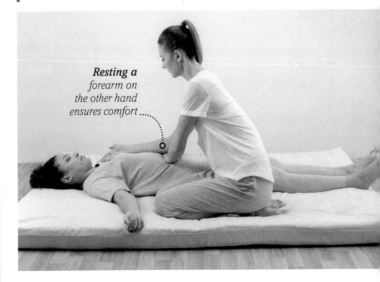

Resting a forearm on the other hand ensures comfort

▲ **The side of the forearm** can be used to access a long section of a meridian—for example, along the midline meridian on the upper body. Here, the arm is turned outward to open up the lungs. The forearm is used in a similar way on large areas such as the back.

CONTINUED ▶

SHIATSU *continued*

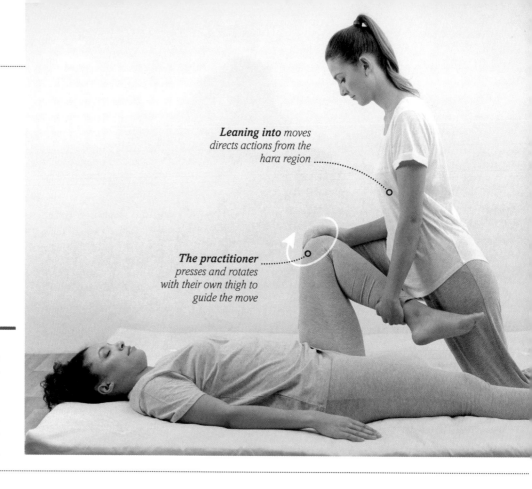

Leaning into moves directs actions from the hara region

The practitioner presses and rotates with their own thigh to guide the move

HIP ROTATOR

Many meridians pass ▶ through the hips so energy can become easily blocked in this area. This guided rotating action opens the hips so that energy can flow smoothly through the body.

SIDE-LYING

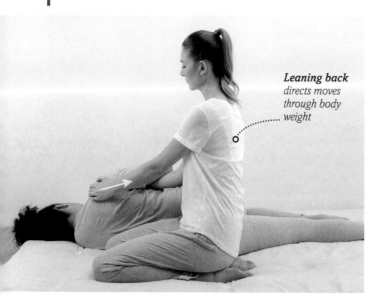

Leaning back directs moves through body weight

▲ **Placing the receiver** on their side gives access to the shoulders from the floor and is also ideal in pregnancy. From here, the practitioner can use their body weight to pull back and rotate the shoulder joint, and can also work on meridian points.

PALMING

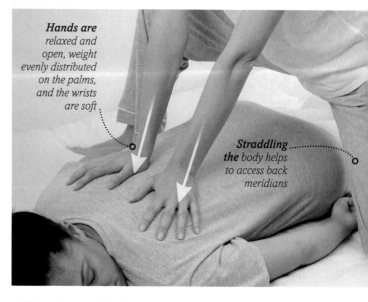

Hands are relaxed and open, weight evenly distributed on the palms, and the wrists are soft

Straddling the body helps to access back meridians

▲ **The palms** provide a large surface area, used to apply pressure all over the body. Again, body weight is used to sink into the move and transfer energy, providing a healing touch that calms, balances, and eases discomfort.

ANCHORING AND CIRCLING

This grounding technique can be used while working on the leg meridians. Here, one hand rests on the sacrum while the other travels down a leg meridian (in this case, working on water elements to remove tension), stopping to access a pressure point in the ankle before traveling to the end of the meridian at a point in the foot. ▼

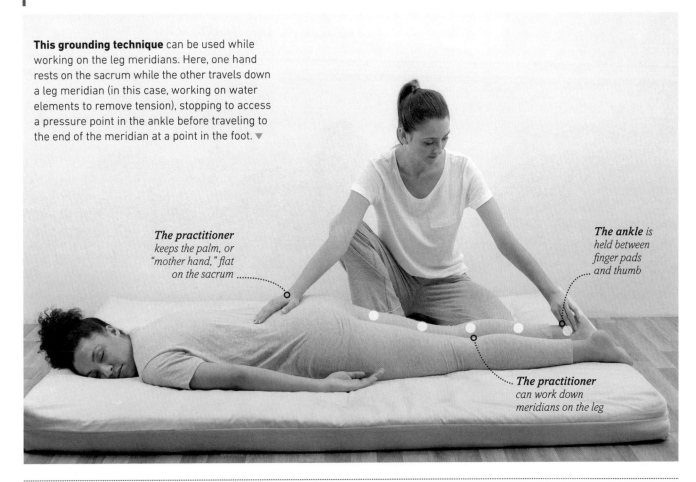

The practitioner keeps the palm, or "mother hand," flat on the sacrum

The ankle is held between finger pads and thumb

The practitioner can work down meridians on the leg

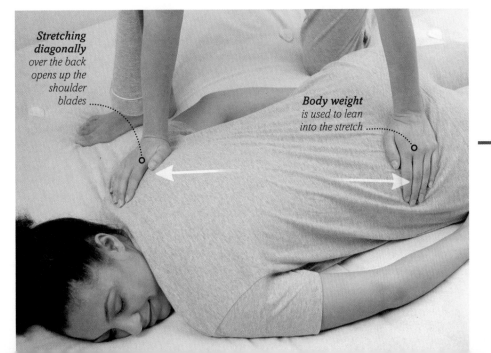

Stretching diagonally over the back opens up the shoulder blades

Body weight is used to lean into the stretch

— STRETCHING

◄ **Stretching can be** done easily over clothes and is used instead of Swedish effleurage and petrissage to release tension. Rocking techniques are also used in this way. As well as easing areas of tension, stretches also help to open up meridians.

KEY FACTS

ESSENCE	TECHNIQUES	BENEFITS
The treatment of tender areas of skin to improve health in another part of the body.	A variety of hand techniques apply pressure to wider areas or specific points.	This noninvasive treatment helps promote mental and physical health.

MASSAGE SPECIALTIES
REFLEXOLOGY

The concept of healing via the feet can be seen in many ancient cultures. Pictographs in the tomb of Ankhmahor, an ancient Egyptian physician dating from around 2400 BCE, depict the treatment of hands and feet, and there is evidence of feet being treated in ancient cultures such as in China, Japan, and India. These ideas have evolved into the various forms of reflexology used today. In the 1890s, an English physiologist, Sir Henry Head, researched the connection between tender areas of skin and diseased organs that he believed to be served by nerves from the same part of the spine. This early work paved the way for the idea of body zones that has developed into today's practice of reflexology.

HOW DOES REFLEXOLOGY WORK?

Reflexology applies pressure to reflex areas, usually on the feet and hands, to achieve health benefits throughout the body. The aim is to restore balance within the body, in turn promoting better overall physical and emotional health while also focusing on the treatment of specific internal organs in the body where problems are identified.

There are various styles of reflexology, many of which focus on the feet, but some also work on the hands, ears, and face. What links all of these styles is the precise application of pressure to a particular area of skin using knowledge of the reflexology zones, which in turn is believed to have a beneficial effect on another part of the body.

Some reflexology practitioners believe that the interaction with the body's nervous system through the stimulation of pressure-sensing nerves causes the response elsewhere in the body. Other practitioners work on the principle that certain points activate different meridians—the energy-carrying channels in the body—helping remove blockages to energy so that it can flow freely throughout the body.

Reflexology treats a range of common complaints and is also used to promote fertility, optimize health during pregnancy, and assist labor. Its noninvasive nature also makes it a useful therapy for children and the elderly and frail.

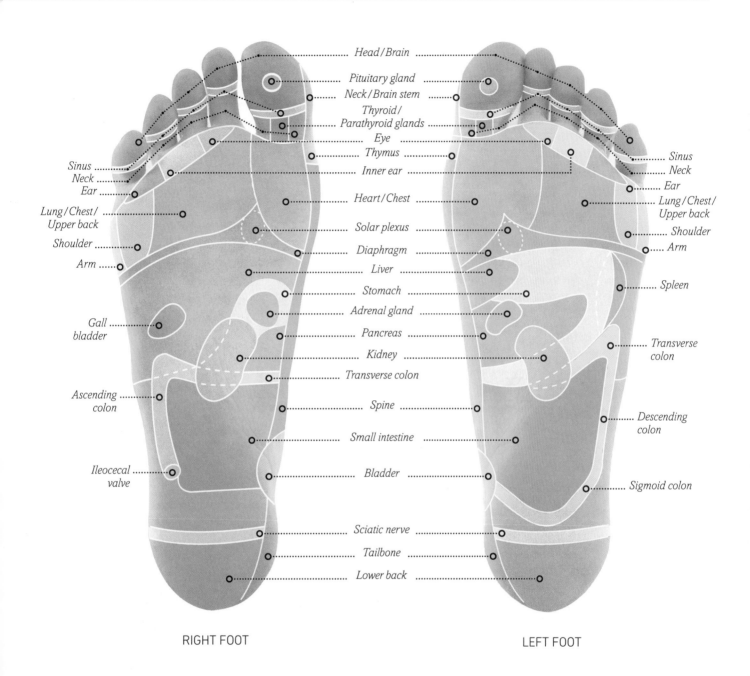

Head/Brain

Pituitary gland

Neck/Brain stem

Thyroid/
Parathyroid glands

Eye

Thymus

Inner ear

Heart/Chest

Solar plexus

Diaphragm

Liver

Stomach

Adrenal gland

Pancreas

Kidney

Transverse colon

Spine

Small intestine

Bladder

Sciatic nerve

Tailbone

Lower back

Sinus
Neck
Ear

Lung/Chest/
Upper back

Shoulder

Arm

Gall
bladder

Ascending
colon

Ileocecal
valve

Sinus
Neck
Ear

Lung/Chest/
Upper back

Shoulder

Arm

Spleen

Transverse
colon

Descending
colon

Sigmoid colon

RIGHT FOOT

LEFT FOOT

▲ FOOT MAP

A reflexology map of the feet indicates reflex areas
that connect to different areas or organs in the
body. Working on a reflex promotes health in the
respective part of the body. The map of the right
foot relates to areas on the right side of the body
and the map of the left foot to areas on the left side.

REFLEXOLOGY

Specific reflexology techniques are used to apply pressure both over the whole foot and to focus on a specific point to address particular concerns, using a foot map (or a hand map if working on the hand) as a guide. Relaxation techniques, such as the side-to-side technique shown opposite, are used at the start of a session and in between techniques.

BASIC TECHNIQUES USED:
○ **Static pressure, p.72**
○ **Stretches, p.74**
○ **Rotations, p.76**
○ **Kneading, p.60**
○ **Knuckling, p.58**

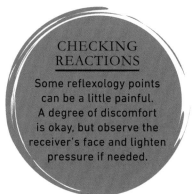

CHECKING REACTIONS

Some reflexology points can be a little painful. A degree of discomfort is okay, but observe the receiver's face and lighten pressure if needed.

THUMB WALKING

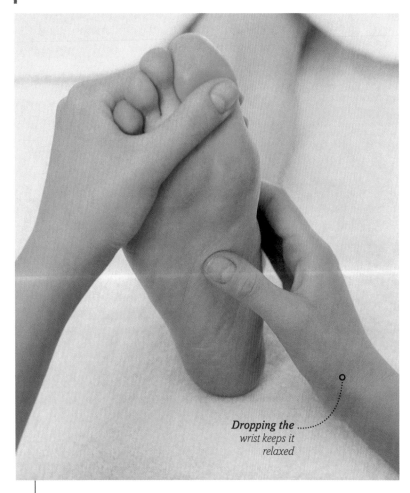

Dropping the wrist keeps it relaxed

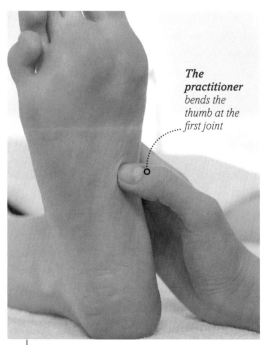

The practitioner bends the thumb at the first joint

① **Thumb walking uses steady pressure** to work over an area on the foot. The practitioner supports the toes in one hand and gently stretches out the sole. The working thumb is then placed on the sole and pressure is exerted with the thumb.

② **The thumb is bent** and then straightened at its first joint to move it along the foot. The practitioner continues to bend and straighten the thumb to "walk" up the sole, gradually moving over an area.

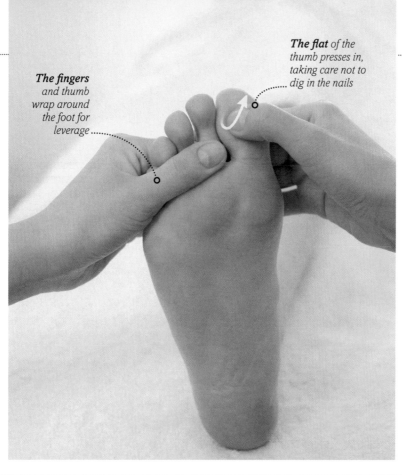

The fingers and thumb wrap around the foot for leverage

The flat of the thumb presses in, taking care not to dig in the nails

— HOOK AND BACK UP

◀ **This technique** works on a specific point to improve health in the corresponding part of the body. The thumb makes a very small, subtle movement here, pressing in deeply to hook the flesh and then pressing the flesh back up.

❙ ROTATION ON A POINT

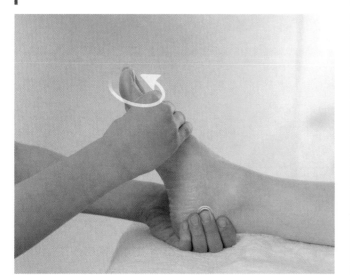

▲ **This works on a specific reflex area**. The middle finger of the hand holding the ankle applies pressure to a point, while the hand at the top of the foot rotates the foot clockwise several times, then counterclockwise. This creates an on-off effect on the reflex point as the foot rotates.

❙ SIDE TO SIDE

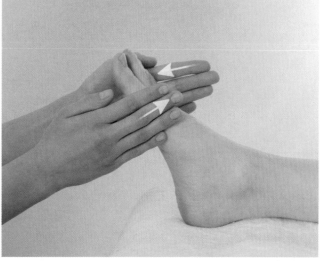

▲ **This relaxation technique**, which moves the foot from side to side between the hands, warms up tissues at the start of a session and is returned to throughout to relax tissues. Other relaxation techniques include gentle pulling to create traction, kneading the sole with the thumbs, and knuckling the sole.

SPECIALTIES

INDIAN HEAD MASSAGE

The tradition of Indian head massage comes from women massaging plant-based oils into their scalp and hair to keep their hair long, strong, and beautiful. Barbers also traditionally offered an invigorating and refreshing scalp massage. The Indian head massage practiced in the West today combines a variety of traditional techniques with massage to other parts of the upper body that typically hold stress, such as the face, neck, shoulders, and arms. It also aims to balance the body's energy, or prana as it is called in Hindi, where interruptions can lead to disease.

KEY FACTS

ESSENCE	TECHNIQUES	BENEFITS
Relaxing and invigorating massage to the upper body, neck, scalp, and face.	Uses basic massage techniques and pressure point work.	A portable treatment that balances energy and releases tension.

HOW DOES INDIAN HEAD MASSAGE WORK?

As well as working on the three upper chakras to rebalance energy and help prana move freely around the body, an Indian head massage practitioner aims to treat many common symptoms associated with stress and working at a computer, such as eye strain, headaches, and neck and shoulder tension. It can also improve overall energy levels and help concentration, leaving the receiver with a feeling of enhanced well-being.

In the West, Indian head massage is usually done without any oil while the receiver is clothed. The only equipment that is required is a comfortable, low-back chair for the receiver to sit in while the practitioner stands to treat them. This easily transportable and convenient treatment can be used in a variety of settings, such as in the workplace, at events, and in other public places. Where a massage is carried out in a public setting, the practitioner may wish to find a means to create a degree of privacy, such as erecting a screen or setting up in a meeting room.

Various massage techniques are used during Indian head massage, including friction, kneading, effleurage, percussion, and working on pressure points over the head. The practitioner works gently and rhythmically yet firmly to help reduce muscular tension and stress levels while also leaving the receiver feeling energized and refreshed.

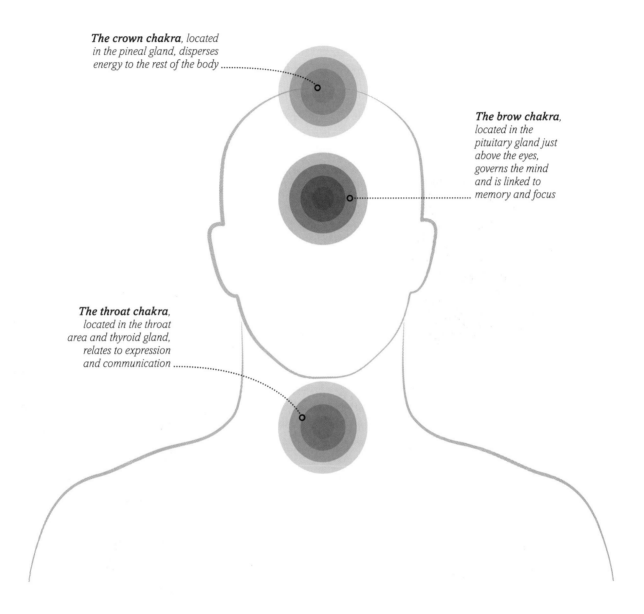

The crown chakra, *located in the pineal gland, disperses energy to the rest of the body*

The brow chakra, *located in the pituitary gland just above the eyes, governs the mind and is linked to memory and focus*

The throat chakra, *located in the throat area and thyroid gland, relates to expression and communication*

▲ **THE CHAKRAS**
The body has seven chakras that relate to specific organs and glands. When balanced, energy flow and health is optimal. Indian head massage works on the three higher ones to enhance energy flow.

INDIAN HEAD MASSAGE

This invigorating head massage both relaxes and energizes. Various techniques are used to relieve muscular tension, including friction, kneading, and pressure point work. No oil is used and the receiver remains dressed. Starting on the shoulders and upper body releases tension here before moving to the neck, scalp, and face.

BASIC AND OTHER TECHNIQUES USED:
- Deep strokes, p.52
- Pressure, p.72
- Kneading, p.60
- Trigger point therapy, p.130
- Slide and glide, p.44
- Vibrations, p.68

RELEASING TENSION IN THE BACK

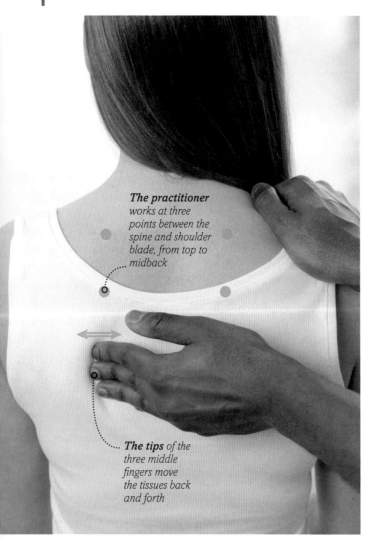

The practitioner works at three points between the spine and shoulder blade, from top to midback

The tips of the three middle fingers move the tissues back and forth

▲ **Friction releases** superficial muscles under the skin. The practitioner supports one shoulder while moving the muscles between the spine and opposite shoulder blade back and forth.

RELAXING THE TRAPEZIUS

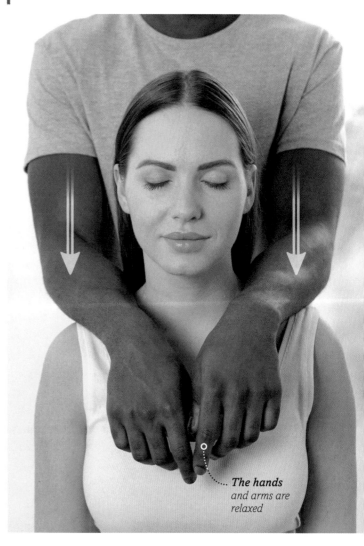

The hands and arms are relaxed

▲ **The forearms** apply pressure to the upper trapezius muscles, where tension is often held. The practitioner leans in, using their body weight and checking that the receiver is comfortable.

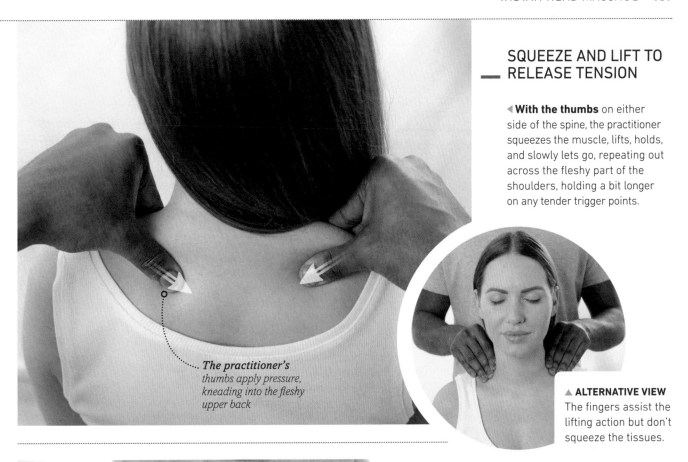

SQUEEZE AND LIFT TO RELEASE TENSION

◀ **With the thumbs** on either side of the spine, the practitioner squeezes the muscle, lifts, holds, and slowly lets go, repeating out across the fleshy part of the shoulders, holding a bit longer on any tender trigger points.

The practitioner's thumbs apply pressure, kneading into the fleshy upper back

▲ **ALTERNATIVE VIEW**
The fingers assist the lifting action but don't squeeze the tissues.

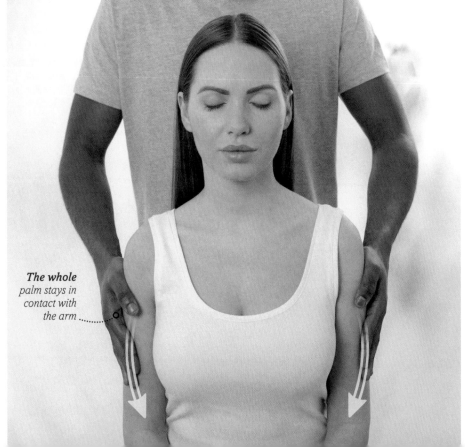

ARM EFFLEURAGE

◀ **The practitioner** places their hands at the top of the arms and strokes down to just above the elbows, applying moderate pressure and repeating this several times. The muscles of the arms are warmed and relaxed a little more with each stroke.

The whole palm stays in contact with the arm

CONTINUED ▶

INDIAN HEAD MASSAGE *continued*

NECK KNEADING

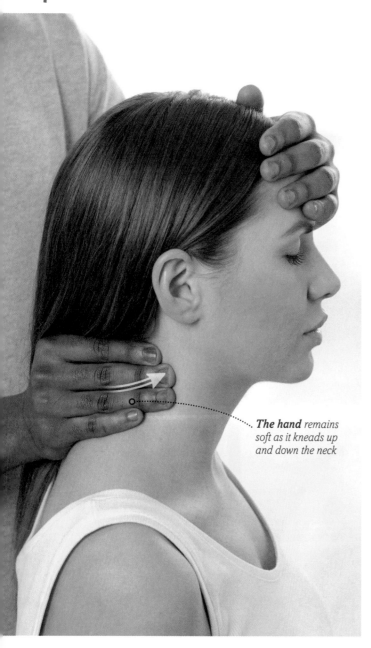

The hand remains soft as it kneads up and down the neck

▲ **The practitioner** supports the forehead with one hand while kneading the neck with the other hand, using the pads of the fingers and thumb and swapping hands to work on both sides of the neck.

"WINDSHIELD WIPER"

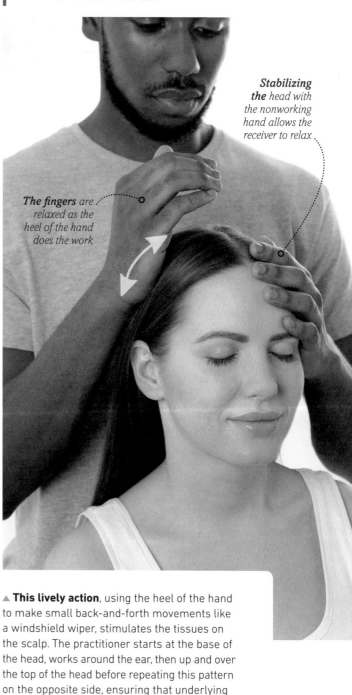

Stabilizing the head with the nonworking hand allows the receiver to relax

The fingers are relaxed as the heel of the hand does the work

▲ **This lively action**, using the heel of the hand to make small back-and-forth movements like a windshield wiper, stimulates the tissues on the scalp. The practitioner starts at the base of the head, works around the ear, then up and over the top of the head before repeating this pattern on the opposite side, ensuring that underlying tissues, and not just the hair, are moving.

HEAD SQUEEZE

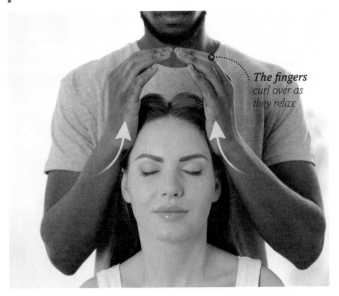

The fingers curl over as they relax

▲ **To release scalp tension**, the practitioner places the heels of the hands on either side of the head, then gently squeezes in to lift the tissues slightly and briefly hold, repeating this around the scalp.

HAIR TUG

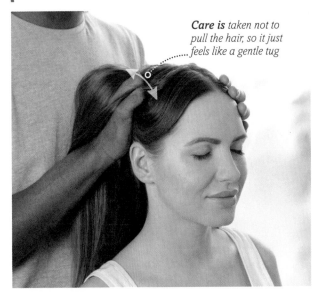

Care is taken not to pull the hair, so it just feels like a gentle tug

▲ **This deeply relaxing action** releases tension in the scalp muscles and invigorates the tissues. The fingers hold the hair close to the roots, then move back and forth to move the scalp, working over the head.

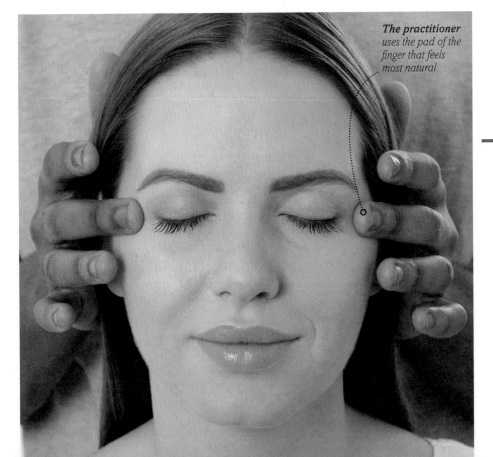

The practitioner uses the pad of the finger that feels most natural

WORKING FACIAL PRESSURE POINTS

◄ **Working on** facial pressure points (see p.171) relaxes muscles. The practitioner starts at the forehead and works down around the eyes (avoiding the eyelids and eyes) and nose, using light pressure. Each point is held for a couple of seconds before moving slowly to the next one, keeping pressure constant. Points on either side of the nose and nostril may be held longer and light friction used to help with sinus issues.

KEY FACTS

ESSENCE	TECHNIQUES	BENEFITS
A noninvasive approach to younger- and more vibrant-looking skin.	Gentle touch moves excess lymphatic fluids; vigorous touch exfoliates skin.	Reduces the appearance of wrinkles and sagging and eases puffiness.

SPECIALTIES

FACIAL REJUVENATION

The practice of facial rejuvenation originates from Indian Ayurvedic medicine (see p.138), the ancient healing system that evolved around 5,000 years ago. Massage is an important element within Ayurvedic practice to maintain health and beauty. Facial rejuvenation massages the face alone, drawing on Ayurvedic principles. The practice, sometimes referred to as a "natural facelift," is a noninvasive approach to looking and feeling younger, using massage and pressure point techniques to improve the health of the skin and muscles of the face and to reduce feelings of emotional stress.

HOW DOES FACIAL REJUVENATION WORK?

Facial rejuvenation includes both gentle and some more vigorous facial massage, carried out without using any oil on completely clean skin. During the massage, the Ayurvedic pressure, or pulse, points are stimulated to relieve tension in the face and jaw, and techniques are used to balance energy through the higher chakras, the energy centers of the body (see p.164). Working on the chakras helps encourage the flow of the body's natural energy, known as prana in Hindi. In Ayurveda, blockages in the flow of this energy cause symptoms of pain, fatigue, and disease.

The practitioner uses repetitive finger movements over wrinkles in the skin, as well as techniques to release tension in the muscles of the face, neck, and scalp, helping both to smooth away fine lines on the face and improve the elasticity of the underlying connective tissue and skin.

Gentle massage techniques are used to help flush away excess lymphatic fluids and reduce puffiness in the face, while the more vigorous movements naturally exfoliate, sloughing off the dead cells to revitalize and rejuvenate the skin.

As well as being a popular treatment for improving the appearance of skin, facial rejuvenation can also be used to relieve localized problems such as sinusitis and headaches, to promote relaxation to tackle concerns such as insomnia, and to alleviate the symptoms of stress.

PRESSURE POINT MAP
This facial map shows the order in which pressure points can be worked on during facial rejuvenation. The key below indicates how groups of points can help relieve different physical symptoms. ▼

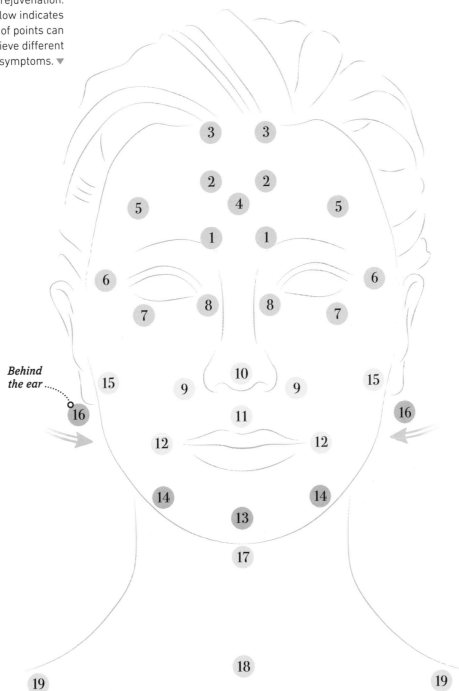

Behind the ear

KEY

Forehead points: *boost concentration and relax muscles to improve elasticity.*

Eye points: *relieve eye strain.*

Nose, mouth, and cheek points: *help decongest blocked sinuses.*

Jaw points: *relieve headaches caused by jaw tension and some types of earache.*

Neck points: *these points, on bony areas, promote relaxation.*

FACIAL REJUVENATION

BASIC TECHNIQUES USED:
○ **Effleurage, p.40**

This uses deeply relaxing effleurage to remove tension in the jaw and face, clear sinuses, and boost lymphatic drainage, as well as stimulating moves to break down sticky collagen to smooth out lines and rejuvenate skin. No oil is used, and skin should be clean. Also, the practice should be avoided with Botox fillers. Some key techniques are shown here, with full training needed to master the practice.

▌WORKING ON PRESSURE POINTS

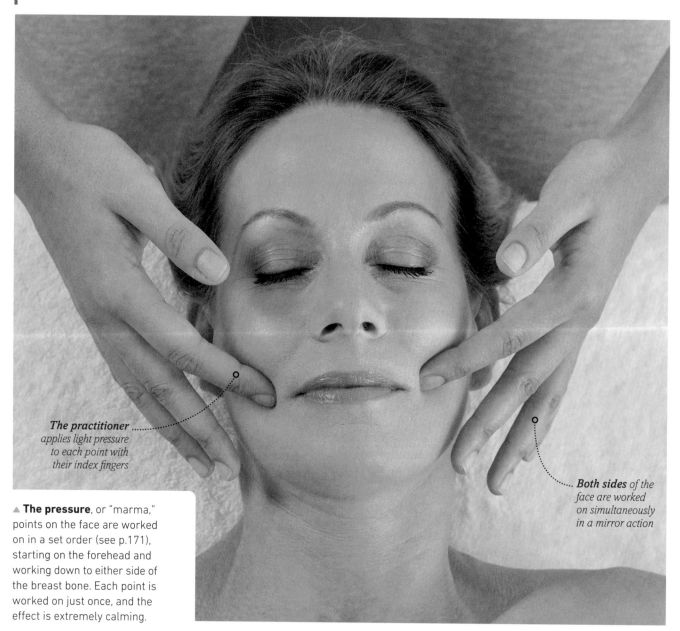

The practitioner applies light pressure to each point with their index fingers

Both sides of the face are worked on simultaneously in a mirror action

▲ **The pressure**, or "marma," points on the face are worked on in a set order (see p.171), starting on the forehead and working down to either side of the breast bone. Each point is worked on just once, and the effect is extremely calming.

RELAXING THE FACE

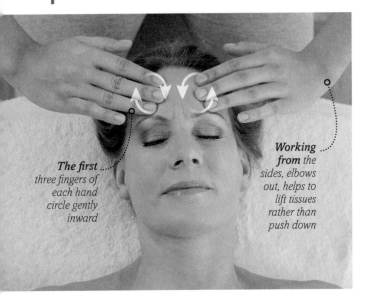

The first three fingers of each hand circle gently inward

Working from the sides, elbows out, helps to lift tissues rather than push down

▲ **Circling** over the face, starting at the top and working down, releases the fascia and relaxes the facial muscles. This action works into the muscle, not just the skin, gradually building depth.

EXFOLIATING

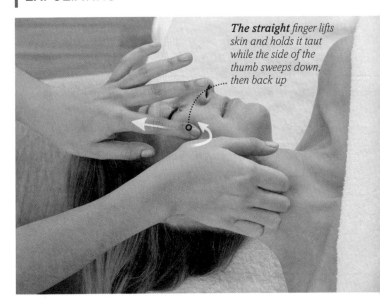

The straight finger lifts skin and holds it taut while the side of the thumb sweeps down, then back up

▲ **Lifting the muscle** up with a finger, then sweeping tissues down with the side of the thumb, removes dead cells to "resurface" the skin. As the move is repeated, the skin becomes smoother.

LINE SMOOTHING

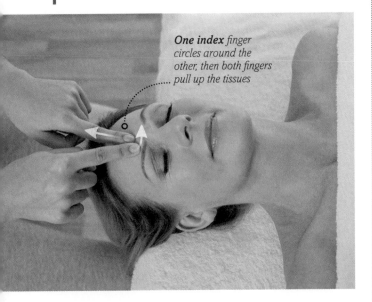

One index finger circles around the other, then both fingers pull up the tissues

▲ **Small, precise** moves break down "set" tissues to smooth lines. The fingers pummel and pull tissues, going from top to bottom on both sides of the face, varying pressure depending on the fragility of skin.

LIFTING

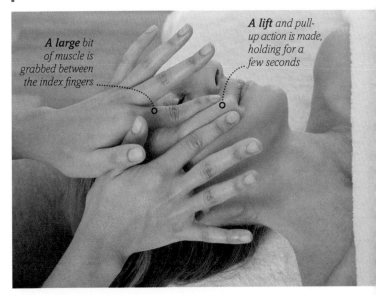

A large bit of muscle is grabbed between the index fingers

A lift and pull-up action is made, holding for a few seconds

▲ **This strong, lifting** technique is done toward the end of a session, when tissues are warmed up. It is done on fleshier areas and on the jawbone (not the forehead) to relax muscle and make it feel lifted.

TAILORING TREATMENTS

There is no such thing as a one-size-fits-all massage treatment. Each person has his or her own particular needs, and these may change from day to day. Part of the skill of a therapist is to listen and assess these needs, then to tailor a massage accordingly, building in adaptations to a full-body massage or perhaps just focusing on particular areas within a shorter time frame. Here, guidance is given on how to develop an assessment-based treatment plan to focus your massage. Suggestions for tailoring treatments for a range of situations are also provided—from balancing energy to improving well-being; to relieving the symptoms for a range of common complaints; to tailoring a massage to suit the needs of particular client groups. A brief baby massage sequence for parents to enjoy is also included.

KEY

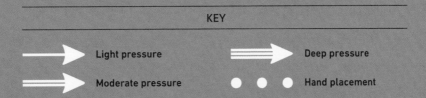

Light pressure

Moderate pressure

Deep pressure

Hand placement

MAKING A TREATMENT PLAN

The aim of massage therapy is to help optimize health, using oils to support treatments if desired. Devising a clear treatment plan tailored to an individual's needs helps you work with intention and purpose. Even those seeking a one-off massage will benefit from the clarification of goals that a treatment plan offers. Bear in mind that health concerns can evolve over time, so treatment plans need to adapt accordingly to meet these changing needs.

ASSESSING NEEDS

Someone requesting a massage may present with a particular health issue or reason for seeking the treatment. Adopting a problem-solving approach, working together to establish what the person's specific needs are and what the goals of the treatment should be, will help you work systematically and holistically to decide on the treatment objectives. Actively involving the receiver in their treatment plan from the start helps form a mutually beneficial and trusting partnership.

An initial consultation may be slightly longer so that you can ask questions about general health and medical history to help you formulate a plan. You should also identify any contraindications now, such as broken skin or an infection (see p.36), and bear in mind that there may be times when it is necessary to advise the person to visit a more specialized practitioner. The key is to approach each person as an individual with their own specific needs. The following prompts can guide you as you make a treatment plan:

VISUAL ASSESSMENT
A quick visual check can flag up areas of concern at the start of a treatment. ▼

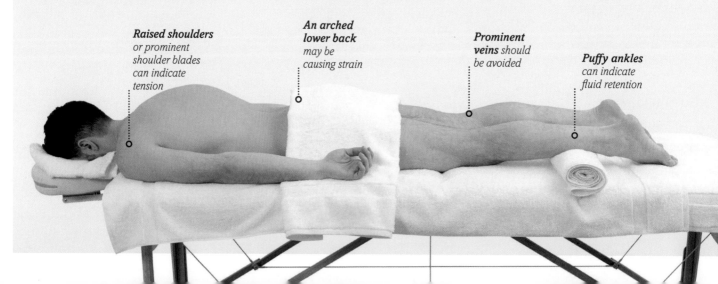

Raised shoulders *or prominent shoulder blades can indicate tension*

An arched lower back *may be causing strain*

Prominent veins *should be avoided*

Puffy ankles *can indicate fluid retention*

"A clear treatment plan will help focus your massage, allowing you to work with intention and clarifying your goals."

- **Establish the main reason** for the massage treatment. Is it to aid relaxation and increase well-being, or is there a more specific aim—for example, to increase energy levels, reduce local pain, or tackle symptoms of stress?
- **Ask about any symptoms and their location.** For example, is there tension or stiffness in the upper back, neck, and shoulders, or are symptoms more general, such as a pervasive feeling of chronic tiredness?
- **Check the frequency of a symptom** and whether it is an acute or chronic concern. This can inform your treatment, and you may find you need to focus on one area of the body at a time at different sessions.
- **Check for triggers**. Is there a particular time or event that comes to mind when the receiver first felt a symptom?
- **Discuss the impact** of a symptom on daily life, bearing in mind that physical symptoms may have an emotional impact and vice versa.
- **Once the receiver is lying** on the massage bed, a quick visual assessment of the body can help you identify areas of concern (see opposite).
- **During the massage**, you may want to assess the effects of the treatment. For example, if there is lower back pain, you might work on this area first, then return to it later to see if there is a noticeable softening of the tissues. You may also need to assess inflammation. To do this, apply enough pressure to cause mild discomfort and hold for 10 seconds. If the discomfort increases, the area should be avoided during the massage treatment.

SHARED GOALS

Exploring areas of concern together helps focus treatment for both parties, bringing the goals of both practitioner and receiver into alignment.

GOING FORWARD

Take notes before and after a treatment so you have a record of what has been discussed and can follow the pattern of treatment and any improvements. Notes can also be useful if you need to share information with a specialist. At the end of the massage, suggest a treatment plan for going forward. Explain your aims for each session and manage expectations so that the receiver is aware of what you can and cannot do.

TAILORING TREATMENTS

MASSAGE THERAPY FOR WELL-BEING

Everyday demands can leave us feeling stressed and overwhelmed, unable to step back and unwind, or, equally, depleted of energy and lackluster. Aromatherapy massage is a powerful tool for rebalancing and grounding, providing a space to step away and allow the therapy of touch, coupled with therapeutic essential oils, to relax body and mind. The release of tension in the muscles and the stimulation to the circulatory and lymphatic systems has numerous benefits, helping release stiffness and improve posture, detoxify, focus the mind, and promote relaxation, all of which helps revitalize and recharge.

DE-STRESSING

The aim of all massage is to relax the tissues and release tension. During times of chronic stress, muscles can be particularly tense and the mind clogged. A flowing whole-body massage with tailored essential oils helps the receiver completely unwind, slowing the mind and calming stressful thoughts. Maintaining an even pressure throughout helps ground and calm the receiver. Ensure that pressure is firm enough to help them let go. Spending more time working on the back helps remove tension here, while soothing work on the head and feet can be profoundly relaxing.

BASIC TECHNIQUES USED:
○ **Fan stroke, p.40**
○ **Circle strokes, p.46**
○ **Stretches, p.74**

| RELAXING THE BACK

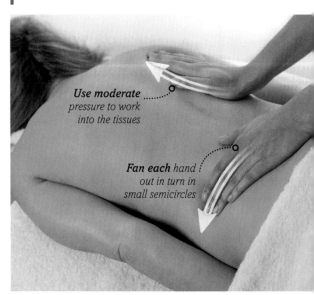

Use moderate pressure to work into the tissues

Fan each hand out in turn in small semicircles

▲ **Effleurage all over the back** at the start of your massage to warm and relax the tissues and help release stickiness in the fascia. Make either small fans up the back, alternating hands, or one large fan.

SOOTHING HEAD CIRCLES

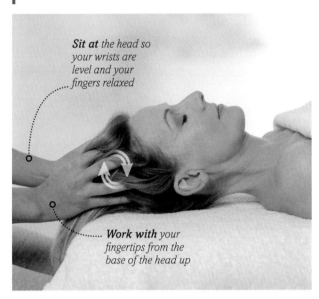

Sit at the head so your wrists are level and your fingers relaxed

Work with your fingertips from the base of the head up

▲ **Circling over the scalp** after the receiver turns over can quickly return them to a relaxed state after being disturbed. Move the tissues under the skin, not just the skin, so the muscles are worked.

RELEASING STRETCH

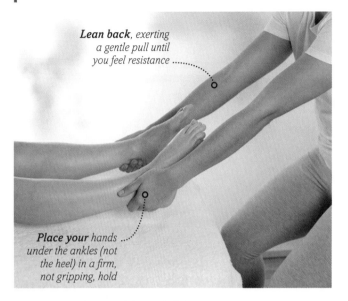

Lean back, exerting a gentle pull until you feel resistance

Place your hands under the ankles (not the heel) in a firm, not gripping, hold

▲ **A leg stretch** toward the end of the massage allows the body to release completely and helps the receiver to feel as though the body has been relaxed from head to toe.

GENTLE NECK PULL

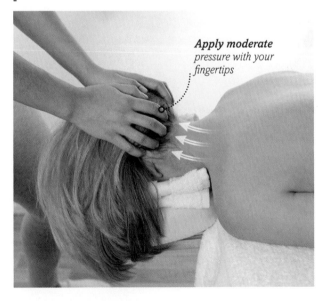

Apply moderate pressure with your fingertips

▲ **For a deeply relaxing finish** to the back, glide your fingertips up the neck, stretching the neck gently, then curl your fingers under the bony occipital ridge and hold for a few moments.

SCALP SELF-MASSAGE

Sit at a table, elbows on the table, and rest your head in your hands as you gently massage the scalp with your fingertips.

Essential oils

Some useful de-stressing oils include:

○ **VETIVER** *to ground and help calm stress-related symptoms.*

○ **PATCHOULI** *for its uplifting and grounding properties, helping counter negative emotions around stress.*

○ **NEROLI** *for balancing and helping ease anxiety.*

PATCHOULI ▶

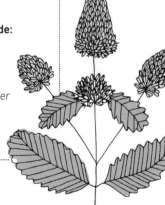

ENERGIZING MASSAGE

Feeling sluggish and de-energized can have multiple causes, from digestive issues to stress, so it's important to try to establish the root cause and tailor your massage if needed. Incorporate plenty of lively petrissage and effleurage into your massage, paying extra attention to the head and feet, where massage can be particularly stimulating.

BASIC TECHNIQUES USED:
○ **Circle strokes, p.46**
○ **Slide and glide, p.44**
○ **Thousand hands, p.42**
○ **Knuckling, p.58**
○ **Percussion, p.64**

STIMULATING HEAD MASSAGE

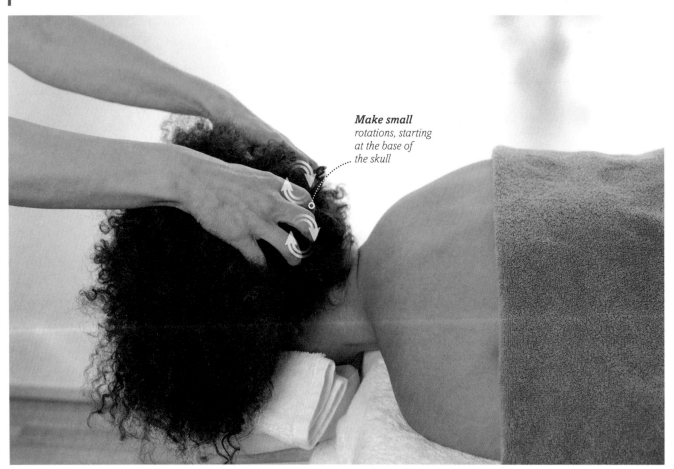

Make small rotations, starting at the base of the skull

▲ **Massaging the head** can feel both relaxing and stimulating. Working on the head at the start of a whole-body massage—before working on the back—can be especially energizing and revitalizing. Use your fingertips to circle over the back of the head, working pretty deeply and quickly—but also taking care not to push the head down into the face hole.

Essential oils

Some helpful oils for energizing include:

○ **BERGAMOT** and **LITSEA CUBEBA**, *which are uplifting and help enhance well-being.*

○ **BLACK PEPPER** *to improve circulation.*

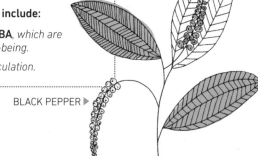

BLACK PEPPER ▶

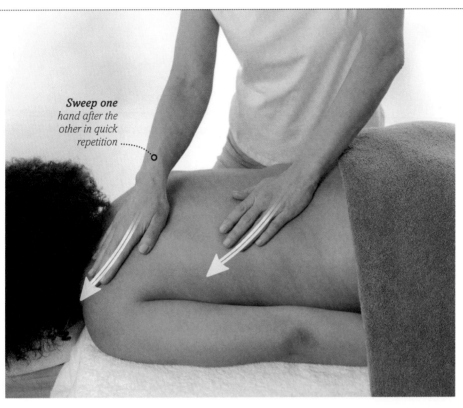

Sweep one hand after the other in quick repetition

GLIDING STROKES

◄ **Give long, sweeping** strokes using the thousand hands technique near the start of the massage to get the blood flowing and flush out waste to energize and cleanse. Work up one side of the back, then repeat on the other side, doing several repetitions on each side until the muscles are warm and relaxed.

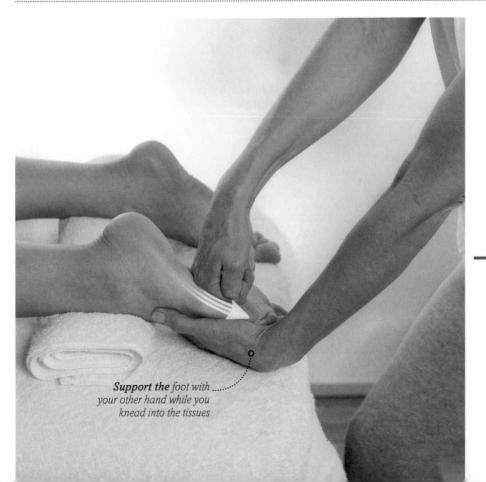

Support the foot with your other hand while you knead into the tissues

DEEP TISSUE WORK ON THE FEET

◄ **If the receiver** is happy to have their feet massaged, this can be particularly stimulating and revitalizing for the whole body. Knuckle over the fleshy areas to wake up the tissues, going pretty deeply to stimulate the circulation. Follow up with some percussion movements over the soles.

TAILORING TREATMENTS

MASSAGE FOR COMMON COMPLAINTS

Massage therapy can help minimize symptoms for a range of common complaints. Used alongside medical treatments, where these are necessary, and lifestyle measures, massaging the body can have profound effects. Techniques stimulate blood flow and warm tissues, helping improve circulatory issues. They also break down adhesions in tissues, in turn relieving stiffness and improving the range of motion, and ground and revitalize, helping increase feelings of well-being and improve mental health. The following pages show how you can focus on and incorporate certain techniques into a massage sequence to relieve symptoms. Basic techniques are used, sometimes combined with disciplines such as trigger point therapy and sports resistance techniques, which can require relevant training.

ARTHRITIS

When massaging someone with arthritis, think about their comfort, whether their mobility is restricted, and if they have referred pain. Check for inflammation, too, and avoid massaging where there is an acute flare-up and/or pain. Work lightly to avoid hurting sensitive tissues. The techniques below focus on the knee and hand, areas commonly affected by arthritis.

BASIC TECHNIQUES USED:
- ○ **Kneading, p.60**
- ○ **Slide and glide, p.44**
- ○ **Circle strokes, p.46**
- ○ **Stretches, p.74**
- ○ **Rotations, p.76**

> ### *Essential oils*
> **Some helpful oils for arthritis include:**
>
> - ○ **ROSEMARY**, **PINE**, *and* **BLACK PEPPER**, *which all have warming and analgesic actions.*

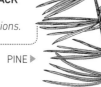

PINE ▶

KNEADING THE KNEE

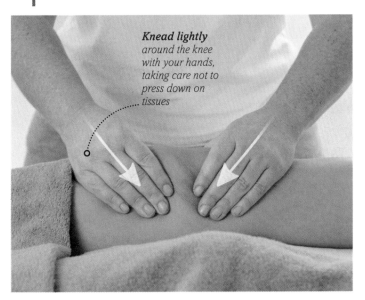

Knead lightly around the knee with your hands, taking care not to press down on tissues

▲ **Gentle kneading** of the fleshy area around the knee helps mobilize the tissues, improving circulation and lymphatic drainage to help reduce inflammation. Effleurage up and down the whole leg before you focus on the knee area.

MASSAGING UNDER THE KNEE

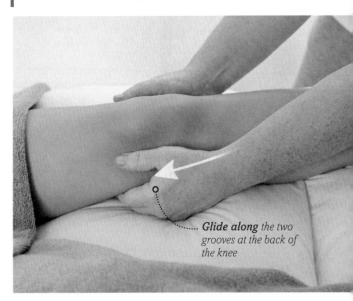

Glide along the two grooves at the back of the knee

▲ **Working under the knee** with the receiver face up lets you loosen tissues without pressing on them and avoids pressure on the top of the knee. In a scooping action, glide your hands along to relax tissues without pressing the back of the knee.

THUMB CIRCLES

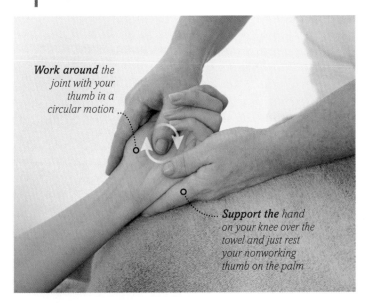

Work around the joint with your thumb in a circular motion

Support the hand on your knee over the towel and just rest your nonworking thumb on the palm

▲ **The hand** is a common site for arthritis. Massage the joints with your thumb to relax tissues and ease stiffness. Keep pressure light, being mindful of the receiver's comfort, going lighter if needed. Give extra time to the base of the thumb joint if especially stiff.

WRIST ROTATION

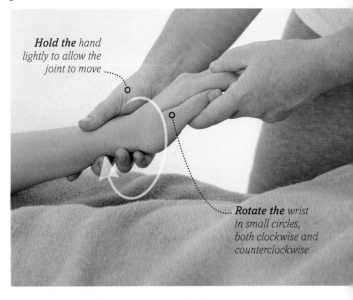

Hold the hand lightly to allow the joint to move

Rotate the wrist in small circles, both clockwise and counterclockwise

▲ **Rotating the wrist** helps loosen this joint, release tension, and ease the stiffness caused by arthritis in the joints of the hand. This passive movement should be done gently, sensing the receiver's range of motion.

BACK PAIN

When assessing back pain, think about where the pain is felt; what makes it better or worse; whether there is a reduced range of motion in any area; and if there is referred pain, for example, traveling down the leg. Effleurage and kneading to warm the tissues can be followed by deeper tissue strokes and trigger point work to release tension and address specific points where pain originates from.

BASIC AND OTHER TECHNIQUES USED:
○ **Deep strokes, p.52**
○ **Pressure, p.72**
○ **Trigger point therapy, p.130**
○ **Slide and glide, p.44**

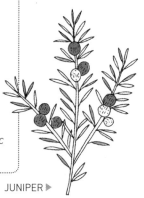

Essential oils

Some helpful oils for back pain include:

○ **MARJORAM** *for its analgesic effect on sore muscles.*

○ **JUNIPER**, *a warming and diuretic oil that helps reduce any swelling of tissues.*

○ **BLACK PEPPER**, *a heating, analgesic oil that improves local circulation.*

JUNIPER ▶

| DEEP EFFLEURAGE ON LOWER BACK

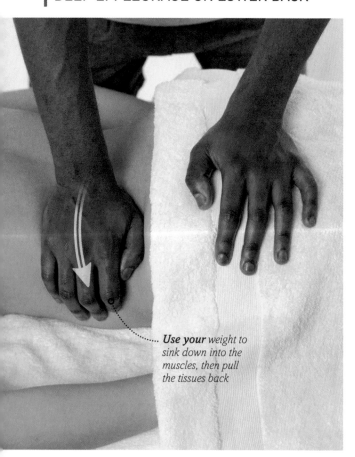

Use your weight to sink down into the muscles, then pull the tissues back

▲ **The lower back**—along the quadratus lumborum muscle—is a common site for pain. After lighter strokes, this deeper effleurage helps the muscle relax, preparing it for deep trigger point work.

| TRIGGER POINT WORK ON LOWER BACK

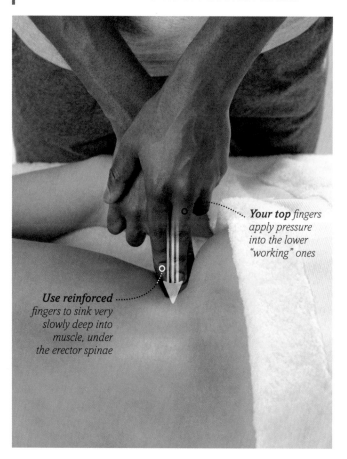

Your top fingers apply pressure into the lower "working" ones

Use reinforced fingers to sink very slowly deep into muscle, under the erector spinae

▲ **The quadratus lumborum** muscle can refer pain into other parts of the back and hips. Once warmed up, work over it to locate possible trigger points, pressing longer on a tender spot until the tissues release.

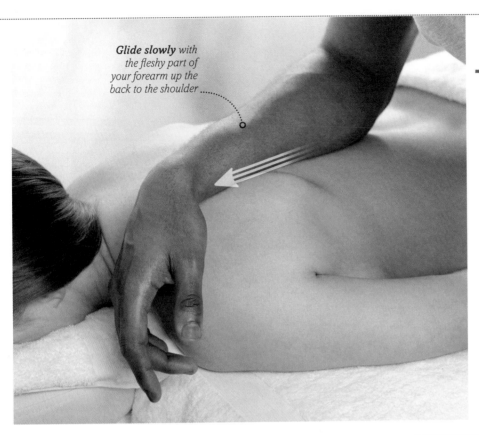

Glide slowly with the fleshy part of your forearm up the back to the shoulder

DEEP FOREARM PRESSURE

◀ **Use your body weight** to apply pressure with your forearm between the scapula and the spine, lunging in to move your arm up. This deep tissue work can reduce pain in the upper back and in other areas, for example, if upper back tension is causing lower back pain.

WORKING ON BACK ERECTOR MUSCLES

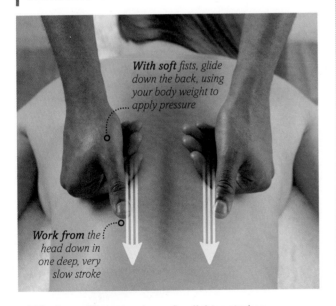

With soft fists, glide down the back, using your body weight to apply pressure

Work from the head down in one deep, very slow stroke

▲ **This deep effleurage**, done after lighter strokes, warms and stretches the erector spinae muscles on either side of the spine. Working down the length of the back lets you address issues in different areas.

RELEASING THE HAMSTRINGS

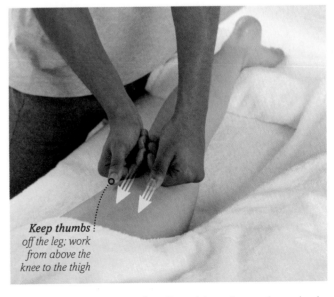

Keep thumbs off the leg; work from above the knee to the thigh

▲ **Tight hamstrings** can pull on the pelvis and cause lower back pain. Applying deep pressure using body weight, after warming effleurage, stretches and warms muscles. The forearm can also be used here. Generally, work on the hamstrings after the back.

NECK TENSION

Tension is commonly held in the neck and can manifest in various ways—for example, causing headaches or restricting movement. Assess how the receiver is affected so you can tailor your massage. Effleurage, stretching, and trigger point work can all be helpful. Always work sensitively with the neck, making movements smooth and slow.

BASIC AND OTHER TECHNIQUES USED:
○ **Slide and glide, p.44**
○ **Stretches, p.74**
○ **Trigger point therapy, p.130**
○ **Knuckling, p.58**

EFFLEURAGING THE NECK

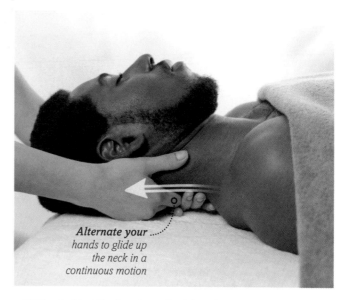

Alternate your hands to glide up the neck in a continuous motion

▲ **Sitting behind the head,** use both hands to stroke up the back of the neck. Keep the hands relaxed, scooping the tissues smoothly without squeezing the flesh. This soothing stroke relaxes muscles before moving to deeper tissue work.

SELF-MASSAGE STRETCH

Sit on one hand to anchor the shoulder. Bring the other hand around the back of the neck onto the same side and gently stretch the neck away from the shoulder.

NECK STRETCH ___

This passive stretch helps ▶ release tension in the upper trapezius muscle. Turn the head away slightly, then put your other hand on the shoulder. Ask the receiver to breathe in, then exhale as you slowly push the shoulder away. Stop at the point of resistance and hold for about 30 seconds, then repeat on the opposite side.

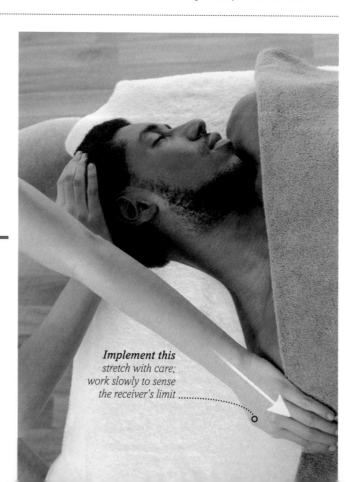

Implement this stretch with care; work slowly to sense the receiver's limit

TRIGGER POINTS: SIDE OF THE NECK

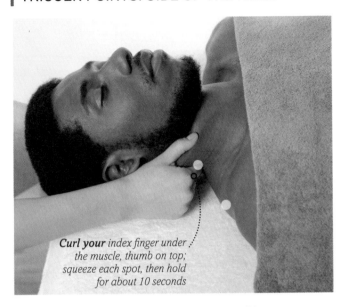

Curl your index finger under the muscle, thumb on top; squeeze each spot, then hold for about 10 seconds

▲ **Trigger point work** on the sternocleidomastoid muscle down the neck can pinpoint the source of headaches. Work down the neck; at a tender point, press down for longer until the tension releases.

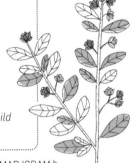

Essential oils

Some helpful oils for muscular tension include:

○ **LAVENDER** *and* **SWEET MARJORAM**, *which have an analgesic effect that can ease muscular pain.*

○ **ROMAN CHAMOMILE** *for its mild anti-inflammatory action.*

SWEET MARJORAM ▶

UPPER TRAPEZIUS MASSAGE

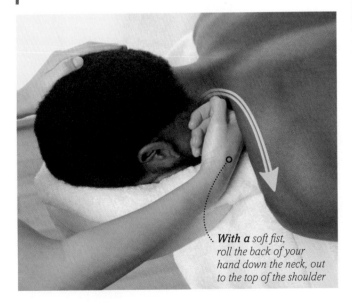

With a soft fist, roll the back of your hand down the neck, out to the top of the shoulder

▲ **Massage around** the upper trapezius and other neck muscles to release chronic tension. This fairly deep introductory stroke warms tissues before trigger point and deeper tissue work.

TRIGGER POINTS: TOP OF THE NECK

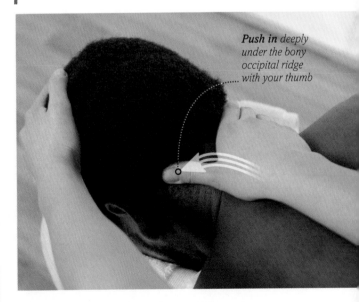

Push in deeply under the bony occipital ridge with your thumb

▲ **Tension in the muscles** at the top of the neck—the suboccipital muscles—can refer pain into the head. Use your thumb to work into this area, feeling for trigger points as you move along.

RESTLESS LEG SYNDROME

This is described as a tingling, crawling sensation in the legs, making it extremely hard to keep the legs still. It can be mild or severe and tends to worsen at night, impacting sleep. There is no known cause, but it can be more common in pregnancy and has been linked to mineral deficiencies and poor circulation. Regular massage incorporating leg stretches and stimulating petrissage can help improve symptoms.

BASIC AND OTHER TECHNIQUES USED:
○ **Stretches, p.74**
○ **Sports massage, p.128**
○ **Wringing, p.56**

CALF STRETCH

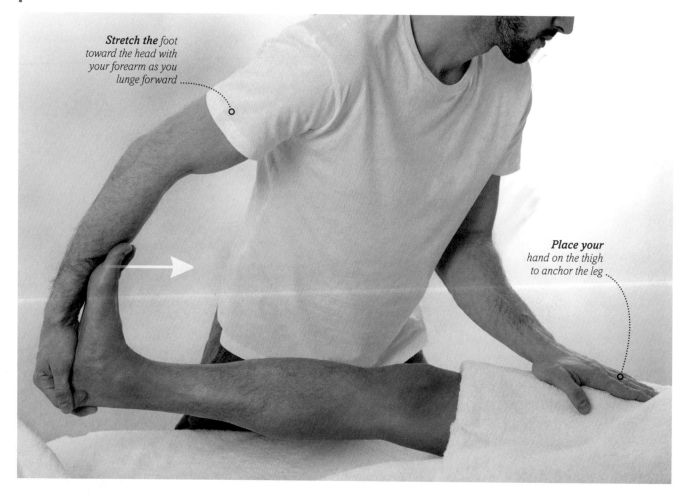

Stretch the foot toward the head with your forearm as you lunge forward .....

Place your hand on the thigh to anchor the leg ...

▲ **Stretching the calf muscles** helps relax the tissues and release tightness in the muscles. This in turn also improves the circulatory and lymphatic systems, helping remove toxins and waste and reduce the intensity of symptoms. The receiver should keep their leg straight, resisting the pressure as you flex the foot back.

Essential oils

Some helpful oils for restless leg syndrome include:

○ **VETIVER**, *which has sedative properties to aid relaxation.*

○ **SWEET MARJORAM** *to stimulate circulation.*

○ **LAVENDER** *for its deeply soothing effect, which promotes relaxation.*

❘ WRINGING THE THIGHS

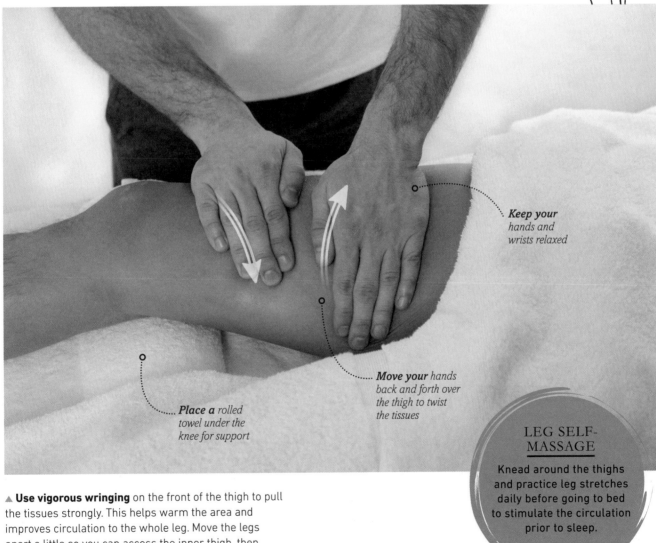

Keep your hands and wrists relaxed

Move your hands back and forth over the thigh to twist the tissues

Place a rolled towel under the knee for support

LEG SELF-MASSAGE

Knead around the thighs and practice leg stretches daily before going to bed to stimulate the circulation prior to sleep.

▲ **Use vigorous wringing** on the front of the thigh to pull the tissues strongly. This helps warm the area and improves circulation to the whole leg. Move the legs apart a little so you can access the inner thigh, then work slowly on the leg closest to you, using just a little oil and moving gradually up and down the quadriceps.

CRAMP

A tendency to cramp—the sudden, painful contraction of a muscle, often in a leg or foot—can have several causes, including muscle strain, dehydration, increased age, or mineral deficiencies. Men are also more prone due to greater muscle mass. A whole-body massage, spending more time on tight leg muscles to release tension, is a good preventative strategy. Work on the thigh first to stimulate lymph drainage into the groin before moving to the calf.

BASIC TECHNIQUES USED:
- Slide and glide, p.44
- Deep strokes, p.52
- Kneading, p.60
- Static pressure, p.72
- Knuckling, p.58

FOOT AND LEG SELF-MASSAGE

When a cramp strikes, use your thumb to stretch and knead tissues on the sole of the foot or knead the calf with your hands.

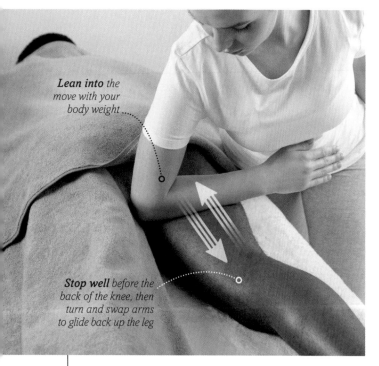

Lean into the move with your body weight

Stop well before the back of the knee, then turn and swap arms to glide back up the leg

(1) **Gliding deeply** with the forearm over the back of the thigh releases tension in tight muscles. Warm the area first with lighter effleurage and petrissage, then work up and down the thigh.

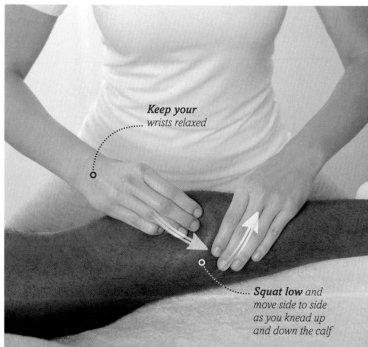

Keep your wrists relaxed

Squat low and move side to side as you knead up and down the calf

(2) **Kneading** up and down the calf after some effleurage relaxes tissues. Sense tense spots and spend a bit longer on these. A deep forearm glide can also be used, but going up only.

Essential oils

Some helpful oils for cramps include:

- **SWEET MARJORAM**, *which is warming and toning for the circulation.*
- **PEPPERMINT** *and* **THYME LINALOOL** *to stimulate the circulation.*

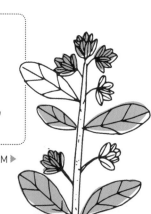

SWEET MARJORAM ▶

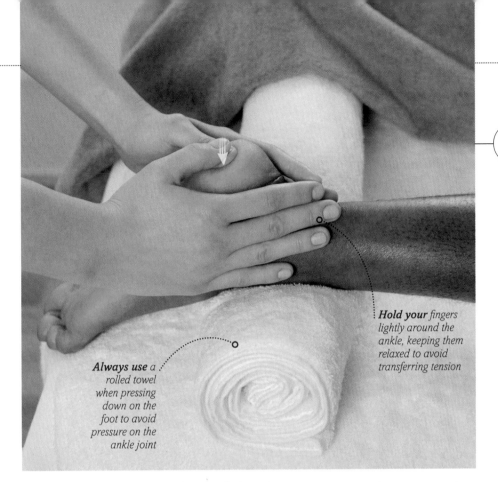

③

The heels can suffer stress from pounding and hold tension that can lead to cramps. Using reinforced thumbs to apply deep pressure over the heel helps break down stickiness in the tissues. Check that the receiver is comfortable with the pressure and go deeper or lighter as needed.

Hold your fingers lightly around the ankle, keeping them relaxed to avoid transferring tension

Always use a rolled towel when pressing down on the foot to avoid pressure on the ankle joint

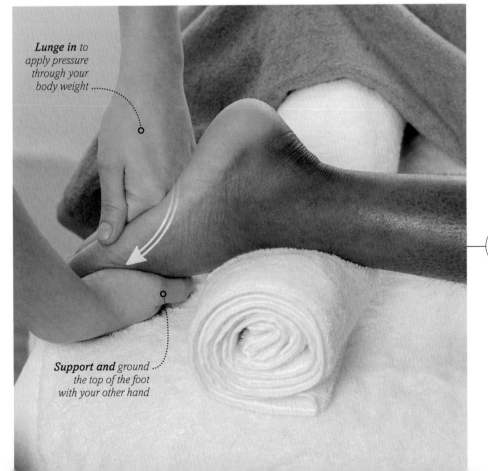

Lunge in to apply pressure through your body weight

④

Work over the sole of the foot with your knuckles, starting at the base of the heel and working all the way down and over the toes. Work down the sole only in this way, and avoid pressing into the heel itself with your knuckles, which can feel uncomfortable.

Support and ground the top of the foot with your other hand

KNEE PAIN

The knee is a complex structure where ligaments and tendons link to bones and muscles in the leg. Pain can be caused by damage to one or more of these structures. With acute pain, massage should be avoided. For chronic pain, it's important to assess the cause. Effleurage and petrissage with essential oils can improve knee health. The stretching techniques here involve more advanced resistance techniques to work on the leg muscles above the knee, where strain can affect the knee.

BASIC AND OTHER TECHNIQUES USED:
○ **Deep strokes, p.52**
○ **Sports massage, p.126**

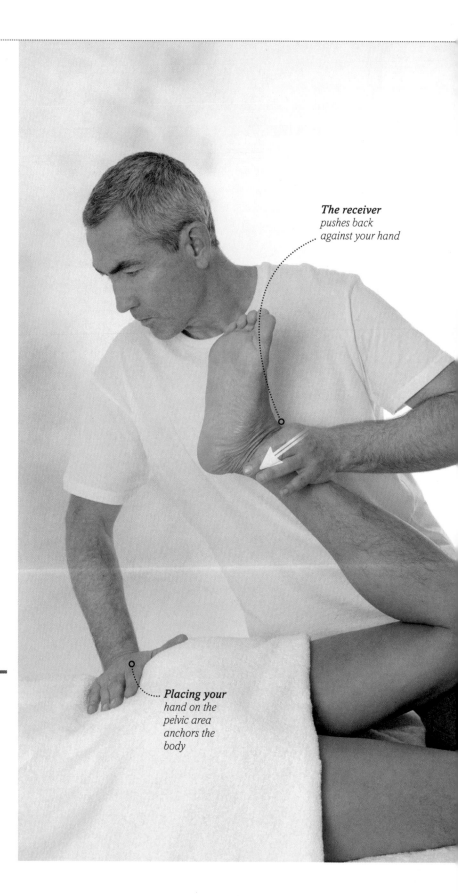

The receiver
pushes back
against your hand

Placing your
hand on the
pelvic area
anchors the
body

QUADRICEPS STRETCH —

Strain in the quadriceps can ▶ radiate down to the knee, so if the quadriceps are tight, stretching and releasing them can help alleviate knee pain. Using your body as anchorage helps stretch the muscle fibers. The thigh is lifted and the leg bent, feeling for the point of resistance while the receiver pushes back, then release before taking it a bit further.

HAMSTRING STRETCH

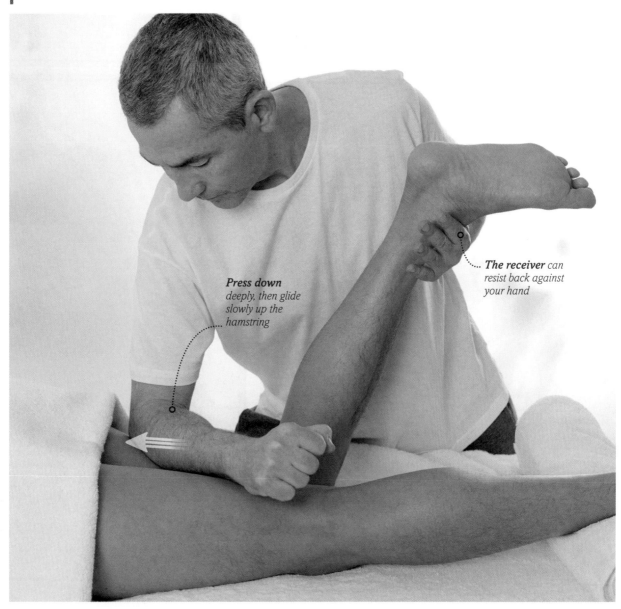

Press down deeply, then glide slowly up the hamstring

The receiver can resist back against your hand

▲ **Working on the hamstring** can help release fibers going into the back of the knee. Your forearm can be used to work deeply into the tissues here, while your other hand moves the lower leg up and down while the receiver resists to help correct imbalances in the muscles.

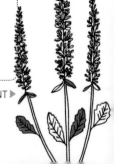

Essential oils

Some helpful oils for knee pain include:

○ **PEPPERMINT** *for stimulating circulation and an analgesic effect.*

○ **GINGER** *and* **BLACK PEPPER**, *which warm the tissues and improve circulation to help soothe localized pain.*

PEPPERMINT ▶

STRAINS AND SPRAINS

A strain involves a tear to a muscle or tendon; a sprain is a torn ligament and is more severe. Both should be treated straight away with the RICE procedure (rest, ice, compression, and elevation). Most massage is avoided in the acute phase of a sprain, as this could damage tissues further, though massage away from the site can boost lymphatic drainage. Other techniques can be done after a few weeks to break down adhesions and aid healing.

BASIC AND OTHER TECHNIQUES USED:
- Slide and glide, p.44
- Circle strokes, p.46
- Sports massage, p.126
- Vibrations, p.68

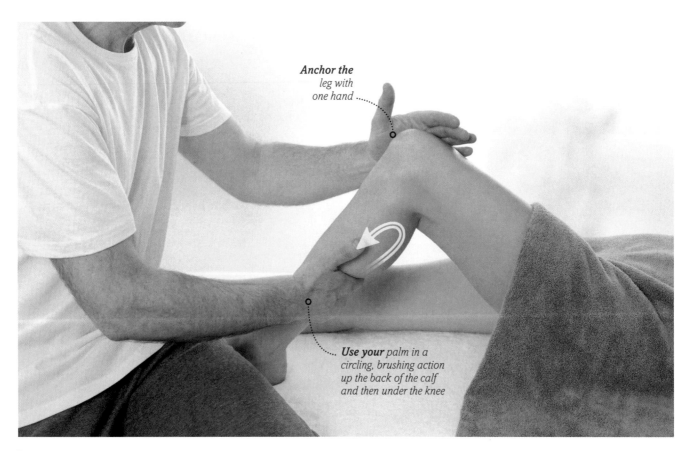

Anchor the leg with one hand

Use your palm in a circling, brushing action up the back of the calf and then under the knee

REDUCING INFLAMMATION

▲ **Light effleurage** can be done away from the injury site in the days after a sprain or strain to drain fluids into the lymph nodes at the back of the knee and into the lymphatic system to ease swelling. Raising the leg to access the lower calf muscles allows the receiver to remain face up to avoid putting pressure on the injury.

Essential oils

Some helpful oils for strains and sprains include:

- **ROMAN CHAMOMILE** *for its anti-inflammatory properties, useful in the acute phase of an injury.*
- **PEPPERMINT** *for its analgesic, cooling effect.*
- **LAVENDER**, *which is soothing and analgesic.*

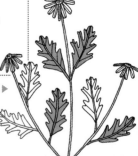

ROMAN CHAMOMILE ▶

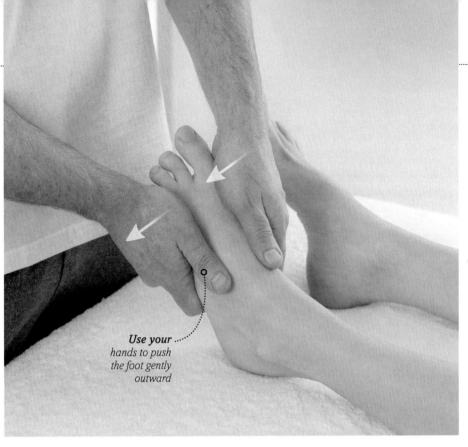

Use your hands to push the foot gently outward

RESISTANCE WORK

◀ **When healing** is underway and there is no swelling, resistance work helps tone the ligaments and restore mobility. As you support the foot and move it outward, the receiver resists, pushing back toward their other foot. The action can be repeated, encouraging the receiver to resist back as far as possible.

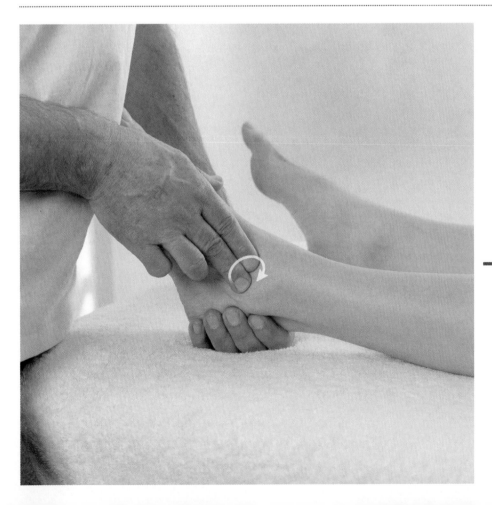

CIRCLING AROUND THE ANKLE BONE

◀ **Gentle friction** across the tendons helps break down adhesions after an injury to promote healing. This is done after a few weeks, when all swelling has subsided. Make tiny circles around the ankle bone, gently vibrating tissues and pressing only lightly, as there is very little flesh here.

FROZEN SHOULDER

Frozen shoulder is a chronic condition whereby connective tissues around the shoulder joint tighten, causing pain and stiffness and limiting movement. The cause isn't always known but can be due to factors such as injury or surgery that keep the arm immobile for some time. Incorporating resistance techniques into your massage helps test the range of motion, while trigger point work can detect the source of pain.

TECHNIQUES USED:
- ○ **Sports massage, p.126**
- ○ **Trigger point therapy, p.130**

CHECKING THE RANGE OF MOTION

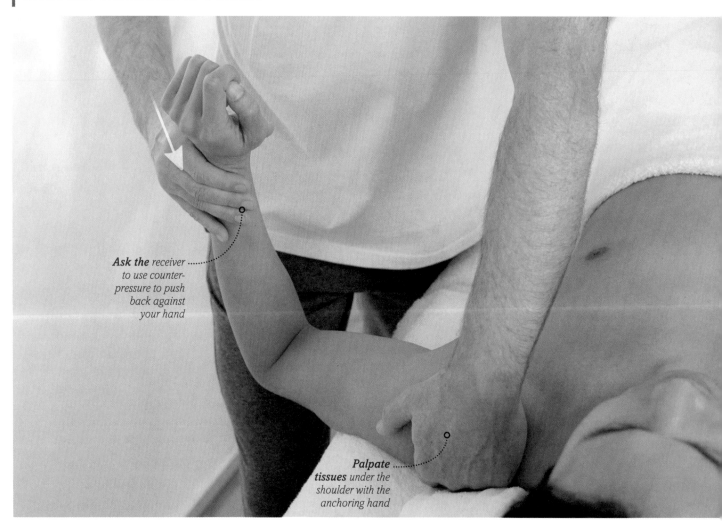

Ask the receiver to use counter-pressure to push back against your hand

Palpate **tissues** *under the shoulder with the anchoring hand*

▲ **Before massaging** the arm and shoulder area, do some resistance work to test restriction in the fibers and carefully extend the range of motion. Hold the arm, pull it toward you, then ask the receiver to push back. Release, then take the arm back a little beyond its point of resistance to test its movement.

Essential oils

Some helpful oils for frozen shoulder include:

○ **GINGER** *to warm tissues and stimulate circulation.*

○ **JUNIPER** *to help soothe muscle pain.*

○ **BLACK PEPPER** *for its heating and analgesic properties and to stimulate the circulation.*

BLACK PEPPER ▶

| TRIGGER POINT AND RESISTANCE WORK

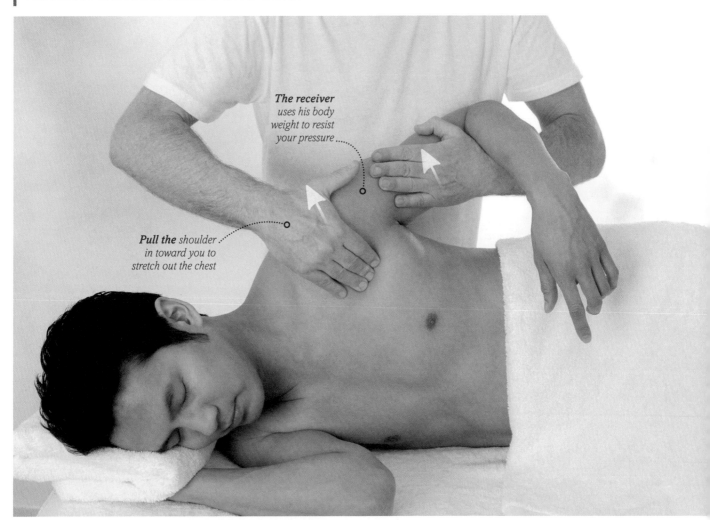

The receiver uses his body weight to resist your pressure

***Pull the** shoulder in toward you to stretch out the chest*

▲ **With the receiver** on his side, palpate the middle of the rotator cuff muscles on the shoulder with your fingers. Press deeply to locate tender trigger points that may be directing pain elsewhere, holding here a bit longer. At the same time, pull the shoulder toward you, asking the receiver to resist to help release tension.

TENNIS ELBOW

Overuse of the lower arm muscles near the elbow joint caused by repetitive movements, sometimes sports-related, can cause pain around the elbow. Initial deep effleurage over the whole arm, working up into the neck, warms the tissues before you target the forearm muscles near the elbow. Here, trigger point therapy can help locate the source of pain, and resistance techniques can test mobility.

BASIC AND OTHER TECHNIQUES USED:
- ○ **Slide and glide, p.44**
- ○ **Trigger point therapy, p.130**
- ○ **Sports massage, p.126**
- ○ **Deep tissue massage, p.114**

❙ TRIGGER POINT AND RESISTANCE WORK

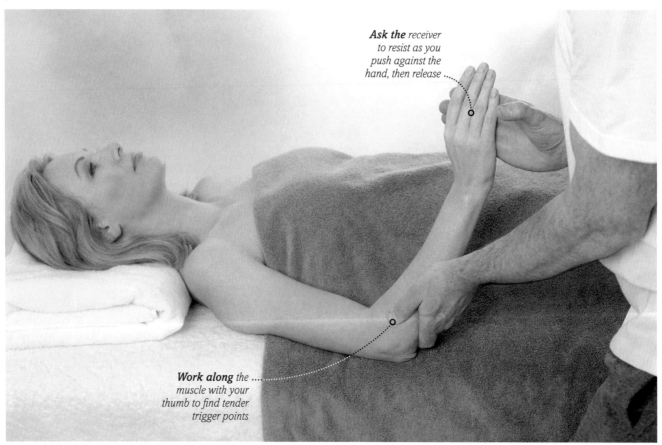

Ask the receiver to resist as you push against the hand, then release ....

Work along the .... *muscle with your thumb to find tender trigger points*

▲ **Trigger point work** combined with resistance techniques locate the source of pain while simultaneously testing and improving the range of motion in the elbow. While working on the trigger point, the receiver can resist pressure in the raised arm to help even out imbalances in the muscle groups and increase the range of motion.

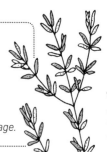

Essential oils

Some helpful oils for tennis elbow include:

- ○ **ROSEMARY** *to stimulate circulation.*
- ○ **THYME LINALOOL** *for its warming properties.*
- ○ **JUNIPER** *to improve circulation and lymphatic drainage.*

THYME LINALOOL ▶

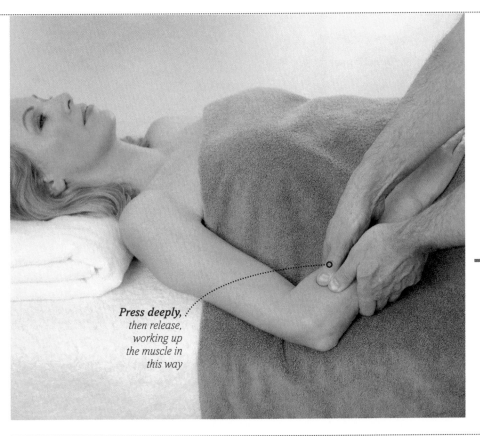

Press deeply, *then release,* *working up* *the muscle in* *this way*

DEEP TISSUE WORK

◂ **Use your thumbs** to work deeply into the tissues on the forearm, working up the extensor muscles here and stopping before the elbow. This helps break adhesions in the tissues and improve local circulation.

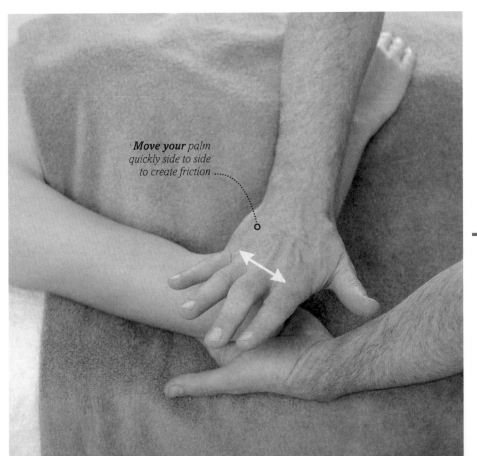

Move your palm *quickly side to side* *to create friction*

ELBOW SELF-MASSAGE

Use your thumb to rub briskly over the elbow, moving up and down to break up stickiness and adhesions in the tissues.

FRICTION

◂ **Damage to**—and overuse of—the elbow causes adhesions to form in the tissues, so lactic acid and waste builds up, resulting in muscle stiffness. Using a rubbing action across the muscle fibers creates friction, helping separate fibers that have stuck together to improve mobility.

REPETITIVE STRAIN INJURY (RSI)

RSI, which includes conditions such as carpal tunnel syndrome and tendonitis, occurs when an action is done repeatedly over long periods of time, such as working at a computer. Muscles tighten in the affected areas, most commonly the upper limbs, restricting circulation and leading to tingling, numbness, and pain. Massage helps stimulate circulation and break down adhesions in tissues. Incorporate the sequence below into your massage to help stretch tissues and improve movement.

BASIC TECHNIQUES USED:
○ **Slide and glide, p.44**
○ **Kneading, p.60**
○ **Circle strokes, p.46**
○ **Shaking, p.68**

▌WARMING THE TISSUES

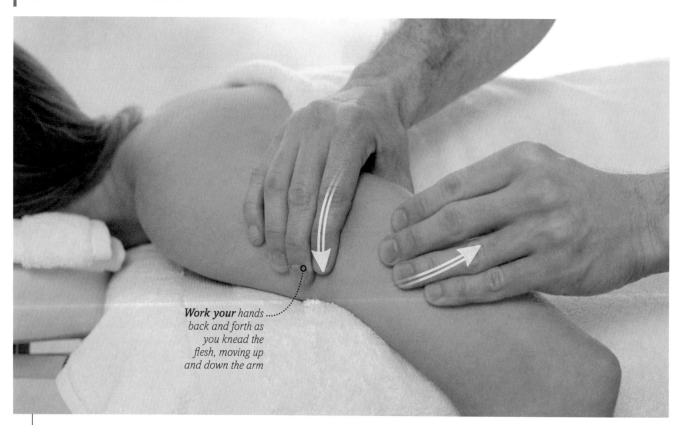

Work your hands back and forth as you knead the flesh, moving up and down the arm

1 **Begin by effleuraging** the whole arm, from the hand to the top of the arm and up around the shoulder, to warm the tissues. Follow with stimulating petrissage kneading on the fleshy upper arm, to help improve circulation here and flush out toxins, in turn stimulating circulation in the whole arm.

Essential oils

Some helpful oils for RSI include:

○ **ROMAN CHAMOMILE**, *which has an anti-inflammatory action that is beneficial for damaged tissues.*

○ **PEPPERMINT** *and* **LAVENDER** *with mild analgesic properties to help reduce pain.*

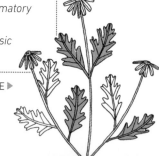

ROMAN CHAMOMILE ▶

GLIDE AND STRETCH MOVEMENT

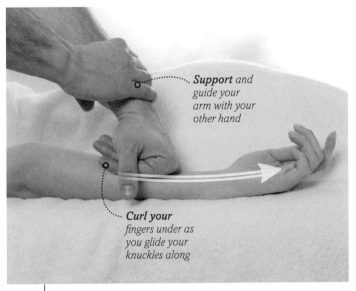

Support and *guide your arm with your other hand*

Curl your fingers under as you glide your knuckles along

2 **Work deeply** into the tissues with a soft fist glide. Glide from shoulder to elbow, then from the elbow down, taking your fist right into the palm to stretch the tissues.

RELEASING TENSION IN THE ELBOW

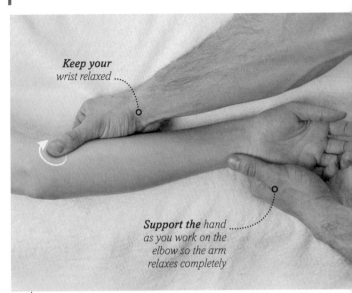

Keep your wrist relaxed

Support the hand as you work on the elbow so the arm relaxes completely

3 **Use your thumb** to circle around—but not on—the elbow joint, helping break down stickiness in the tissues here and reduce inflammation.

WRIST BONE

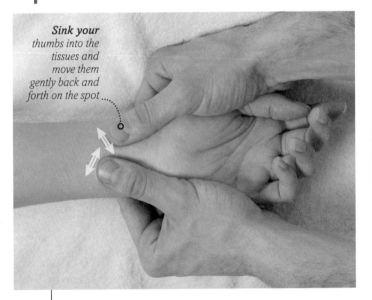

Sink your thumbs into the tissues and move them gently back and forth on the spot

4 **The wrist** is a common site for RSI, as tissues are compressed in this small space. Use your thumbs to make small vibrations to break down sticky spots in the tissues.

PALM STRETCH

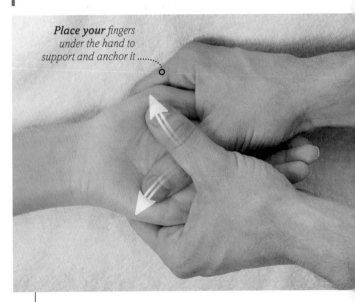

Place your fingers under the hand to support and anchor it

5 **Stretch out the palm** to help release tension here and improve mobility. Glide your thumbs over the palm, using pretty strong pressure to open the palm out.

HEADACHES AND MIGRAINES

Tension in the back, shoulders, neck, and arm caused by factors such as posture, desk work, or stress can all lead to headaches. The causes of migraines aren't always clear, but there can be a tendency to suffer from them. Incorporate the head work here into your massage along with back and shoulder effleurage and deep tissue work to release general tension. Avoid massage in the acute phase of a migraine.

TECHNIQUES USED:
○ **Circular pressure, p.72**

HEAD SOOTHING SELF-MASSAGE

Sit with your elbows on a table. Cup the heels of your hands over the eyes and make small rotations on the scalp with your fingertips.

SCALP ROTATIONS

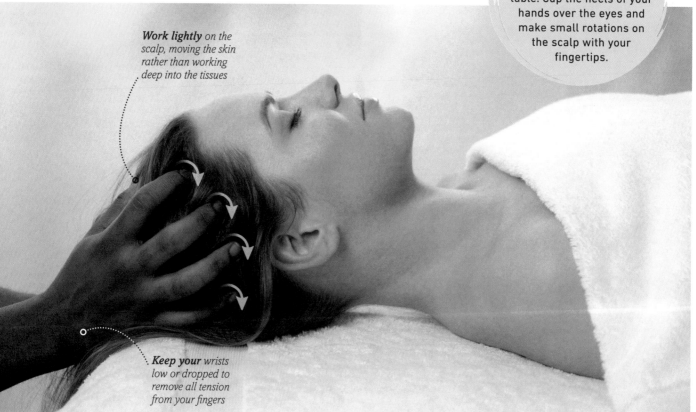

Work lightly on the scalp, moving the skin rather than working deep into the tissues

Keep your wrists low or dropped to remove all tension from your fingers

▲ **Starting off head work** with a soothing scalp massage is a good way to introduce your touch to this part of the body before homing in on specific areas. This general action is beneficial for all types of headaches. Separate your fingers and rest them lightly on the head, then make small on-the-spot rotations, compressing the tissues gently.

Essential oils

Some helpful oils for soothing headaches include:

○ **LAVENDER** *for its analgesic properties.*

○ **PEPPERMINT**, *which is cooling and well-established as a treatment for tension headaches.*

○ **FRANKINCENSE**, *a deeply calming oil that soothes the stress that leads to headaches.*

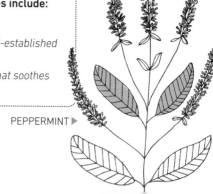

PEPPERMINT ▶

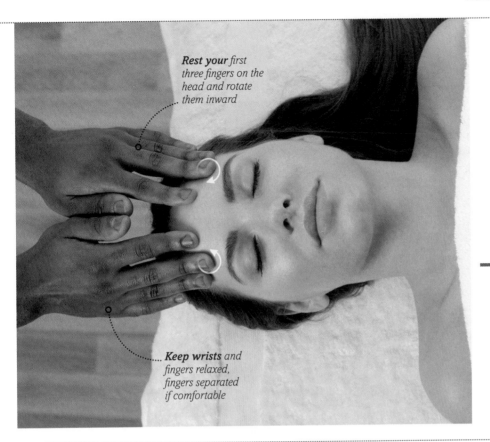

Rest your first three fingers on the head and rotate them inward

Keep wrists and fingers relaxed, fingers separated if comfortable

SOOTHING THE FOREHEAD

◀ **Placing your fingers** on the forehead and circling gently on the spot, applying just a little pressure, helps release both localized and general tension. Work symmetrically on both sides of the forehead, even if the pain or tension is situated mainly on one side.

TEMPLE ROTATIONS

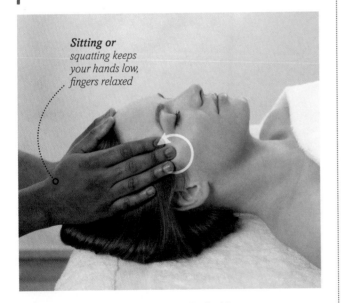

Sitting or squatting keeps your hands low, fingers relaxed

▲ **Pain in the temples** may be soothed with very gentle pressure to this area. Place your first three fingers on each temple and make small rotations, lifting the tissues toward you.

CRANIAL HOLD

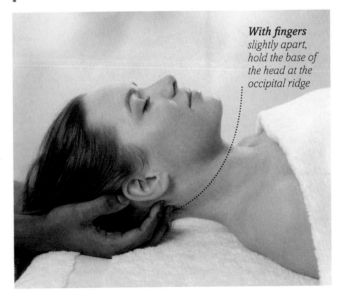

With fingers slightly apart, hold the base of the head at the occipital ridge

▲ **This hold** is typically done at the end of a head massage. Holding the head in this way, letting it sink into your curled fingers so you take its weight, works deeply into the tissues to ease tightness.

SINUSITIS

The sinuses are small cavities behind the cheekbone and forehead. They drain mucus into the nose via tiny channels, but if these become inflamed—usually due to viral infection—the channels close off, causing a painful build-up of mucus. Gentle pressure, going a bit deeper as tissues allow, and sweeping actions help drain mucus from the sinuses to bring relief. If there is fever, massage should be avoided.

BASIC TECHNIQUES USED:
○ **Static pressure, p.72**

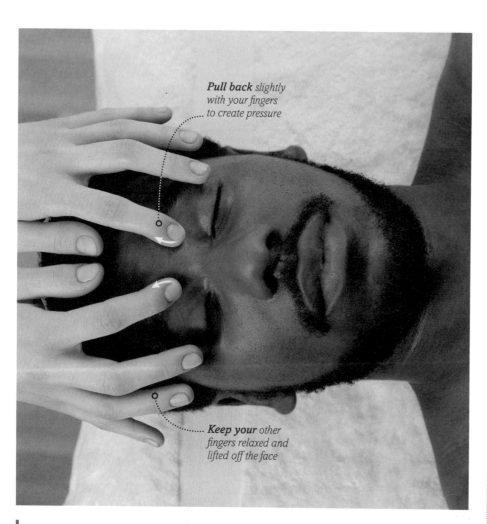

Pull back slightly with your fingers to create pressure

Keep your other fingers relaxed and lifted off the face

DECONGESTING SELF-MASSAGE

Sitting with your elbows on a table, use your index fingers to press on congested areas or your thumbs to press under the eyebrow hook.

EUCALYPTUS GLOBULUS ▶

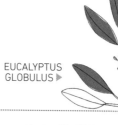

| WORKING ON THE EYEBROWS

▲ **Sitting behind the head,** start at the top of the eyes to relieve sinuses around this area and in the forehead. Place your index fingers in the hook of the eyebrows, then lift slightly, pressing lightly. You can work across pressure points on the brow (see p.171).

Essential oils

Some helpful oils for sinusitis include:

○ **EUCALYPTUS GLOBULUS** *for its mucolytic (mucus-dissolving) effect.*

○ **PEPPERMINT** *for its cooling, mucolytic, and analgesic effect.*

○ **ROSEMARY** *for its stimulating effect on the lymphatic system.*

GENTLE PRESSURE NEXT TO NOSTRILS

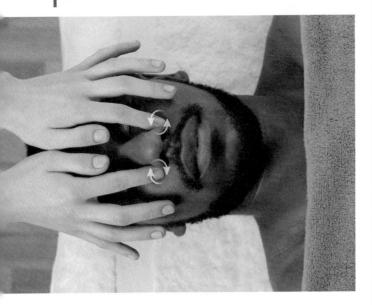

▲ **Work carefully** next to the nostrils, which might be particularly tender. Make small compressions, guided by the receiver on the level of pressure, then either rotate or press down on the spot.

SINUS SWEEP

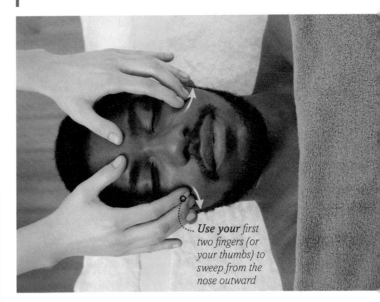

Use your first two fingers (or your thumbs) to sweep from the nose outward

▲ **Make a sweeping action** to move mucus away from congested areas and loosen it. You can do this over the cheekbones, from the nose outward, or over other parts of the face that feel sore.

GENTLE CHEEK COMPRESSIONS

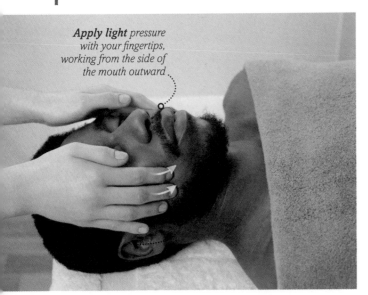

Apply light pressure with your fingertips, working from the side of the mouth outward

▲ **Gently compress the area** next to the mouth to help clear sinuses in this area. Press lightly so you loosen mucus and flush it away rather than compact it. Follow compressions with another sinus sweep.

CHIN DRAINAGE

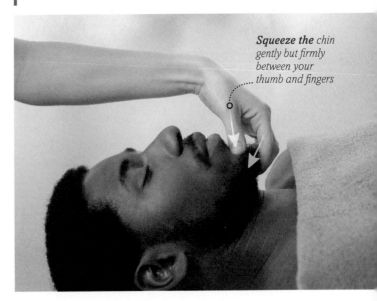

Squeeze the chin gently but firmly between your thumb and fingers

▲ **Release tension in the chin** to aid lymphatic drainage here. Compress the center of the chin with your index finger and thumb, then use both index fingers and thumbs to work in this way down either side of the jaw.

HIGH OR LOW BLOOD PRESSURE

There is no set massage for high or low blood pressure. Where redness in the face indicates very high blood pressure, you may wish to reduce the time the receiver spends face down. Also keep strokes soft, deep, and slow to calm the body, and avoid lively percussion strokes. With low blood pressure, closing grounding techniques help return the receiver to their body; you may also need to assist the receiver off the table if he or she feels dizzy.

BASIC TECHNIQUES USED:
○ **Wringing, p.56**
○ **Stretches, p.74**

HIGH BLOOD PRESSURE: ADAPTED LEG MASSAGE ▬

You can make certain ▶ adjustments to avoid the receiver spending too long lying face down (prone). Raising the leg while the receiver lies face up (supine) allows you to do an adapted wringing action on the calf and back of the thigh, reducing the amount of time the face is compressed.

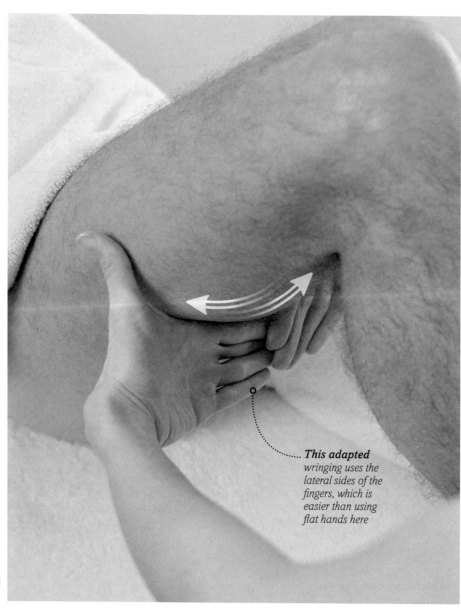

...This adapted wringing uses the lateral sides of the fingers, which is easier than using flat hands here

Essential oils

Some helpful oils for high blood pressure include:

○ **LAVENDER, YLANG YLANG,** and **SWEET MARJORAM,** *which are all sedating and help lower blood pressure.*

Some helpful oils for low blood pressure include:

○ **ROSEMARY, BLACK PEPPER,** and **GINGER,** *all heating oils that stimulate the circulation.*

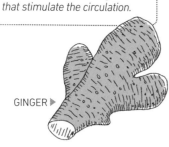

GINGER ▶

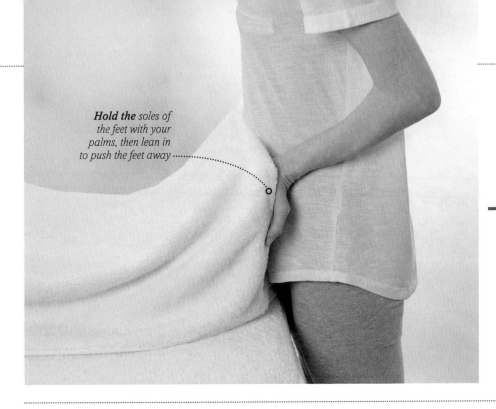

Hold the soles of the feet with your palms, then lean in to push the feet away ⋯⋯

LOW BLOOD PRESSURE: FOOT PUSH

◄ **With low blood pressure**, how you close the massage is important. This firm foot push is strongly grounding. The stretch to the back of the legs and the reassuring pressure readies the receiver mentally and physically to come out of their state of deep relaxation and prepare to get up off the massage bed.

LOW BLOOD PRESSURE: FOOT RUB

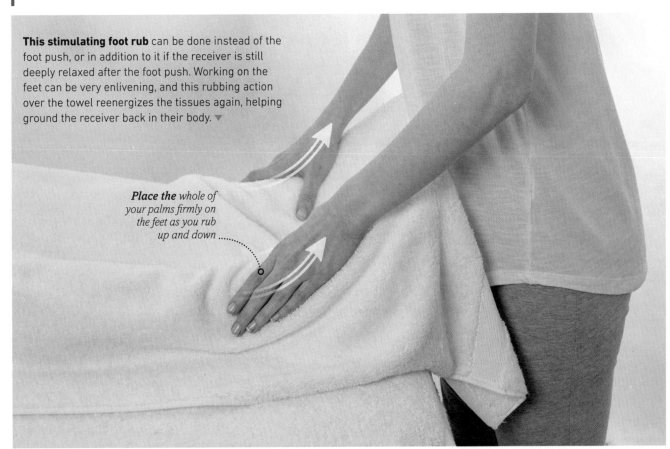

This stimulating foot rub can be done instead of the foot push, or in addition to it if the receiver is still deeply relaxed after the foot push. Working on the feet can be very enlivening, and this rubbing action over the towel reenergizes the tissues again, helping ground the receiver back in their body. ▼

Place the whole of your palms firmly on the feet as you rub up and down ⋯⋯

POOR CIRCULATION

The circulatory system is responsible for moving blood, oxygen, and nutrients around the body. When this isn't working efficiently, it can cause a variety of symptoms, including tingling, cold hands and feet, and sluggish digestion. Possible underlying causes should be investigated, but stimulating massage strokes using some deep effleurage and petrissage techniques in particular can help improve blood flow.

BASIC TECHNIQUES USED:
- ○ **Kneading, p.60**
- ○ **Criss-cross, p.48**
- ○ **Fan stroke, p.40**
- ○ **Circle strokes, p.46**

▌ WORKING ON THE EXTREMITIES

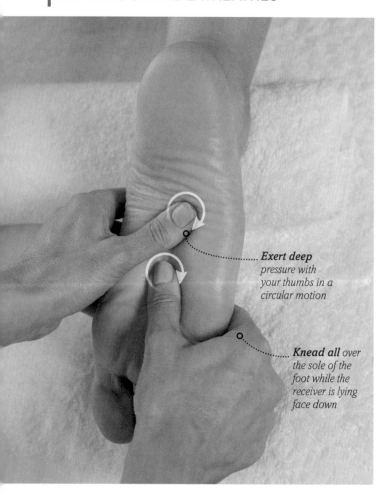

Exert deep pressure with your thumbs in a circular motion

Knead all over the sole of the foot while the receiver is lying face down

▲ **The feet and hands** can become chronically cold when there is sluggish circulation. Kneading with the thumbs helps stimulate the blood flow and warm the tissues. Knead over the sole, then when the receiver has turned over, knead each toe in turn. Similarly, knead the palm of the hand and the fingers.

▌ STIMULATING TISSUES IN THE THIGH

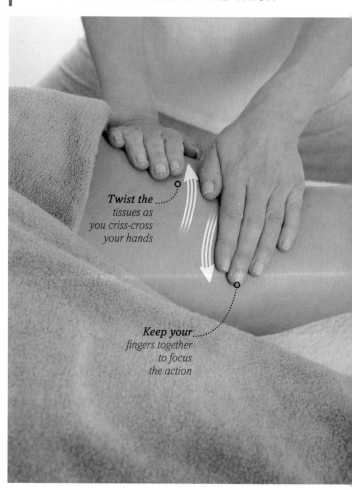

Twist the tissues as you criss-cross your hands

Keep your fingers together to focus the action

▲ **Use a deep effleurage** criss-cross action on the thigh after gliding strokes to warm the tissues thoroughly and encourage blood flow all over the body. Always do deeper work to the thigh before working on the lower leg to drain lymph fluid into the groin, removing blockages and helping stimulate circulation in the whole leg.

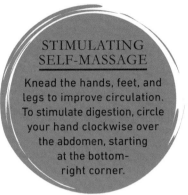

STIMULATING
SELF-MASSAGE

Knead the hands, feet, and legs to improve circulation. To stimulate digestion, circle your hand clockwise over the abdomen, starting at the bottom-right corner.

Essential oils

Some stimulating oils include:

○ **LEMON** and **BLACK PEPPER** *to stimulate sluggish digestion that is linked to poor circulation.*

○ **GINGER**, *a warming and antispasmodic oil.*

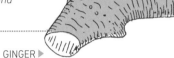

GINGER ▶

STIMULATING DIGESTION

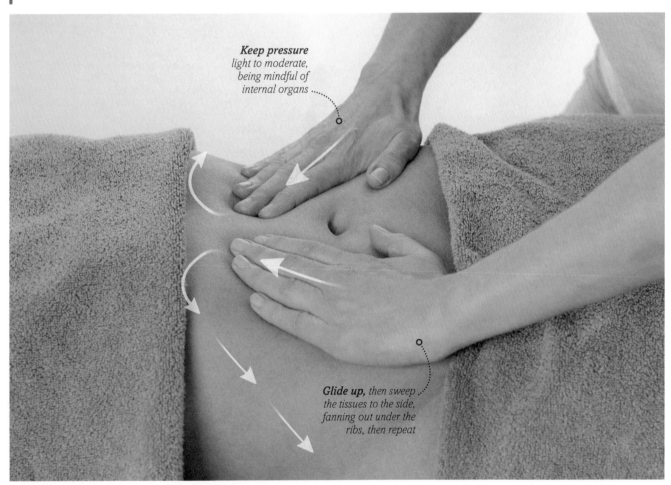

Keep pressure light to moderate, being mindful of internal organs

Glide up, then sweep the tissues to the side, fanning out under the ribs, then repeat

▲ **Poor circulation** can affect digestion, causing it to become sluggish and blocked. An abdominal massage can warm and relax this area, helping stimulate movement in the intestines. Always work slowly and carefully on the abdomen. This fanning stroke stretches and warms the tissues; you can also try a circling action.

VARICOSE VEINS

The improvement to the circulation provided by a whole-body massage can help reduce the severity of varicose veins. However, great care needs to be taken near varicose veins. Assess their severity before you start massaging the leg. If there are just mild threadlike veins, preventative petrissage may be used, but if veins are bulging and prominent, use gentle effleurage only, next to—never over—the affected vein.

BASIC TECHNIQUES USED:
○ **Kneading, p.60**
○ **Slide and glide, p.44**

| PREVENTATIVE PETRISSAGE

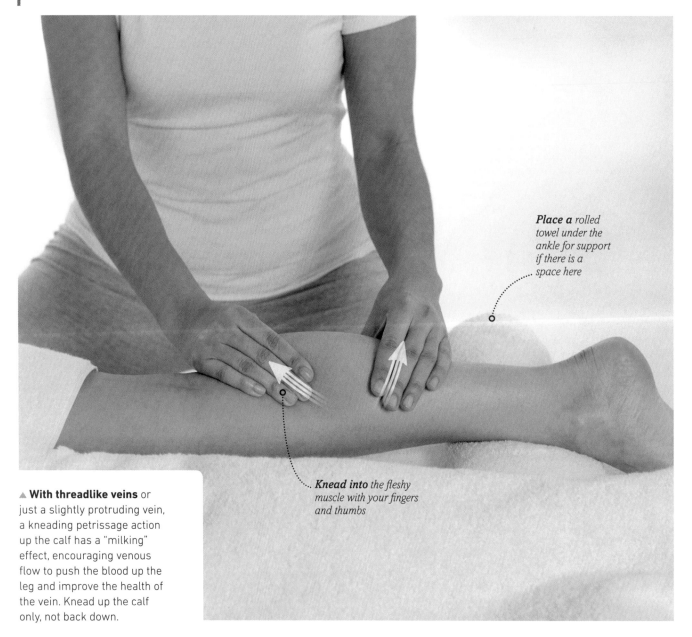

Place a rolled towel under the ankle for support if there is a space here

Knead into the fleshy muscle with your fingers and thumbs

▲ **With threadlike veins** or just a slightly protruding vein, a kneading petrissage action up the calf has a "milking" effect, encouraging venous flow to push the blood up the leg and improve the health of the vein. Knead up the calf only, not back down.

Essential oils

Some helpful oils for varicose veins include:

○ **JUNIPER**, *as its astringent action can help reduce varicose veins.*

○ **LEMON**, *which also has astringent properties that promote lymphatic drainage.*

○ **LAVENDER**, *as it is analgesic, soothing the itchiness and pain of varicose veins.*

LEMON ▼

❙ TREATING WITH EFFLEURAGE

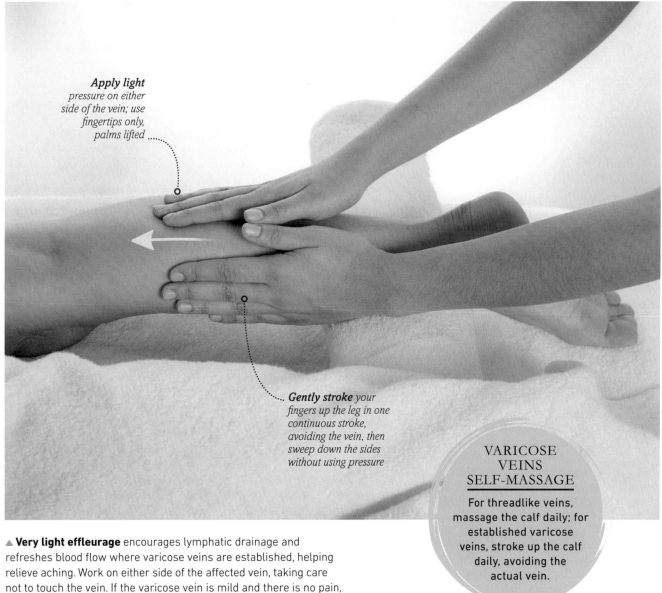

Apply light pressure on either side of the vein; use fingertips only, palms lifted

Gently stroke your fingers up the leg in one continuous stroke, avoiding the vein, then sweep down the sides without using pressure

VARICOSE VEINS SELF-MASSAGE

For threadlike veins, massage the calf daily; for established varicose veins, stroke up the calf daily, avoiding the actual vein.

▲ **Very light effleurage** encourages lymphatic drainage and refreshes blood flow where varicose veins are established, helping relieve aching. Work on either side of the affected vein, taking care not to touch the vein. If the varicose vein is mild and there is no pain, you can effleurage gently over the vein to encourage venous flow.

FLUID RETENTION

A build-up of fluid in the tissues, known as edema, causes localized swelling and can have a number of causes, including poor circulation, being pregnant, and certain medical conditions. When thinking about your approach, take into account any contributing factors. Edema can occur in any part of the body but typically affects the ankles, legs, arms, hands, and face. Focus on a gentle treatment with plenty of soothing effleurage strokes to encourage drainage while avoiding deep pressure on swollen tissues. The techniques below are used to drain fluids from a limb.

BASIC TECHNIQUES USED:
- ○ **Slide and glide, p.44**
- ○ **Thousand hands, p.42**
- ○ **Circle strokes, p.46**

| EFFLEURAGE AROUND THE KNEE

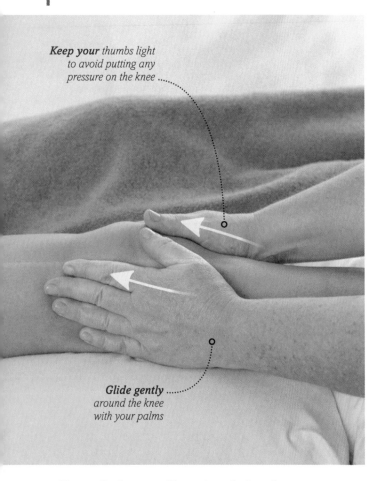

Keep your thumbs light to avoid putting any pressure on the knee .....

Glide gently ..... *around the knee with your palms*

▲ **Elevate the leg** on a pillow to keep it above heart level. Effleurage the whole leg, then give a vigorous thousand hands massage to the thigh before focusing on drainage around the knee. Use gentle pressure, working around—not on—the knee.

| LOWER-LEG EFFLEURAGE

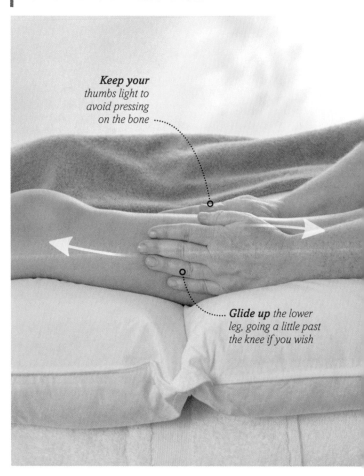

Keep your thumbs light to avoid pressing on the bone .....

..... *Glide up the lower leg, going a little past the knee if you wish*

▲ **Finish** working on the leg by effleuraging up and down the lower leg. Glide up and down with both hands, exerting slightly firmer pressure as you go up to help drain fluids away, then gliding gently back down.

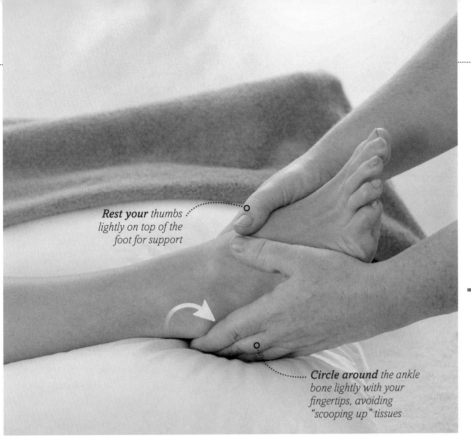

Rest your thumbs lightly on top of the foot for support

Circle around the ankle bone lightly with your fingertips, avoiding "scooping up" tissues

GERANIUM ▶

Essential oils

Some helpful oils for fluid retention include:

○ **JUNIPER, LEMON, AND GERANIUM** *for their detoxifying effects.*

ANKLE CIRCLES

◀ **Fluid can pool** around the ankle bone, making this area particularly swollen and tender. Massaging around the bone helps break up areas of fluid and move waste. When working on swollen ankles, ensure that your touch is extremely light.

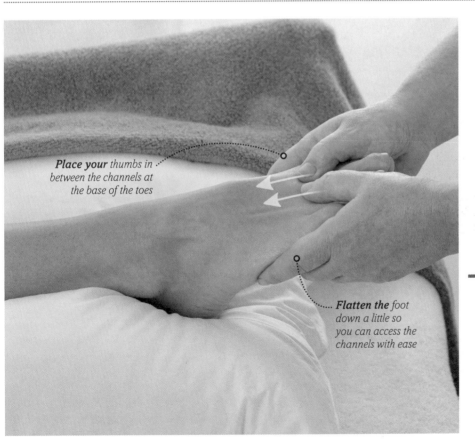

Place your thumbs in between the channels at the base of the toes

Flatten the foot down a little so you can access the channels with ease

SELF-MASSAGE ON THE LEG

Practice regular massage on your thigh and lower leg using gliding strokes, with firmer pressure on the upward stroke.

FOOT "CHANNELING"

◀ **Gliding your thumbs** along the channels between the foot joints helps move excess fluids down the foot and relieve swelling. If fluid retention is chronic, mobility in the feet could be limited, so it's important to work gently and with increased sensitivity. Finish by rotating each toe in turn.

RESPIRATORY COMPLAINTS

Respiratory conditions range from acute infections to chronic complaints. Spend a little more time during your massage on the respiratory area, using stretching, shaking, and percussion techniques to help break up congestion. Work more gently if someone is frail, and with upper respiratory tract congestion, such as sinusitis, make sure you limit the time the receiver spends face down.

BASIC TECHNIQUES USED:
○ **Stretches, p.74**
○ **Rocking, p.70**
○ **Percussion, p.64**
○ **Deep strokes, p.52**

STRETCHING THE RIBCAGE

RIB-OPENING SELF-MASSAGE

Do regular arm stretches, stretching the arm up and over the head to help open up and mobilize the ribs.

Anchor the arm against your body, then pull back with moderate force to achieve an opening stretch

Use your free hand to push the ribs in the opposite direction

▲ **This arm stretch** helps open up the ribcage, stretching out the intercostal muscles to help break up mucus and loosen tightness in the respiratory area. It is particularly beneficial for conditions such as asthma. Squat or lunge to stabilize your position, then repeat the stretch on the opposite side.

Essential oils

Some useful oils for respiratory problems include:

○ **EUCALYPTUS GLOBULUS** and **PINE**, *which are expectorant, mucolytic (dissolving mucus), and have antimicrobial properties to fight infection.*

○ **PEPPERMINT**, *which acts as an expectorant.*

○ **ROMAN CHAMOMILE**, *an anti-inflammatory, sedative, and antispasmodic* and **THYME LINALOOL**, *an antispasmodic—both beneficial for asthma.*

THYME LINALOOL ▶

PULSING THE RIBCAGE

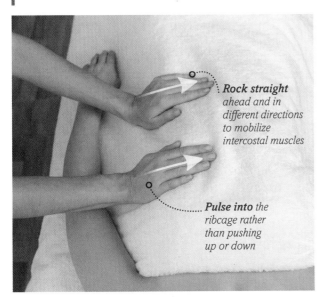

Rock straight ahead and in different directions to mobilize intercostal muscles

Pulse into the ribcage rather than pushing up or down

▲ **A rocking motion** pulses the ribcage to help loosen mucus and decongest. Start gently, then gradually build pressure and work on both sides, spending longer where there is more tightness.

RIBCAGE PERCUSSION

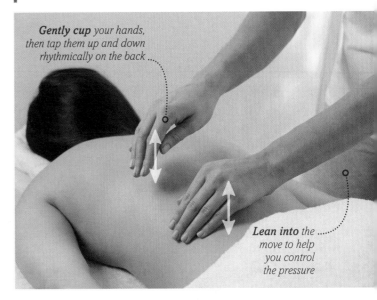

Gently cup your hands, then tap them up and down rhythmically on the back

Lean into the move to help you control the pressure

▲ **Use cupping percussions** over the ribcage on the back. This staccato action helps loosen phlegm and increase blood flow to the area to aid lymph drainage. Work all over the ribs, avoiding the spine.

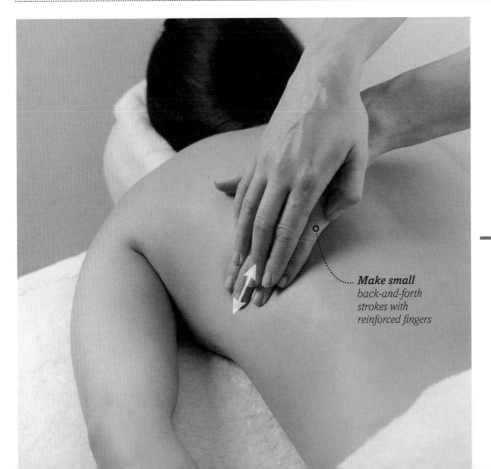

Make small back-and-forth strokes with reinforced fingers

INTERCOSTAL PRESSURE

◀ **More refined**, targeted strokes work into the spaces between the ribs to break up local spots of congestion in the intercostal muscles. Lean in to make this gentle movement, sensing where tissues are especially sticky and adapting the pressure depending on the receiver's level of comfort.

DIGESTIVE COMPLAINTS

Digestive complaints such as constipation, bloating, irritable bowel syndrome (IBS), and acid reflux are often due to poor diet, but stress can also be a factor, so consider the possible causes when thinking about a treatment plan. One common problem, constipation, can benefit from fairly firm abdominal massage to encourage peristalsis (movement of waste along the intestines). Chest-opening techniques that focus on improved posture can also help by ensuring that the digestive organs aren't being compressed by a hunched posture.

BASIC TECHNIQUES USED:
- Fan stroke, p.40
- Circle strokes, p.46
- Kneading, p.60
- Deep strokes, p.52
- Slide and glide, p.44

WARMING EFFLEURAGE

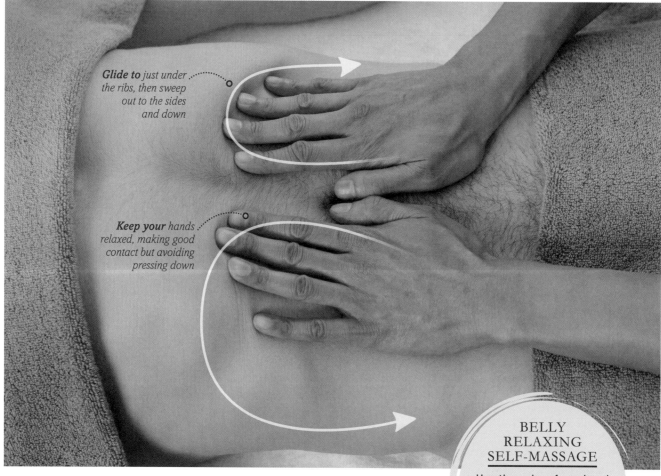

Glide to just under the ribs, then sweep out to the sides and down

Keep your hands relaxed, making good contact but avoiding pressing down

▲ **Working over the whole abdomen** with a large fan stroke or T-stroke warms and relaxes the tissues, helping the muscles to relax. This in turn encourages peristalsis, making this a helpful technique for constipation. Follow this with some circling strokes, working clockwise in the direction of the intestines.

> BELLY RELAXING SELF-MASSAGE
>
> Use the palm of one hand to massage around the abdomen in a clockwise direction using a peppermint essential oil blend.

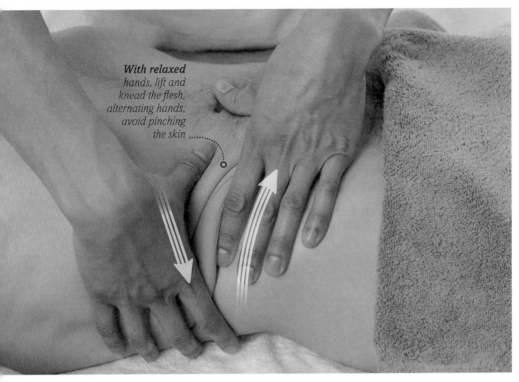

With relaxed hands, lift and knead the flesh, alternating hands; avoid pinching the skin

BELLY KNEADING

◀ **Working between the hips** and ribs, knead the abdomen slowly, increasing depth gradually (as this can be a sensitive area) to stimulate digestion. There is no need to reapply oil after effleurage for this, as you want to get a good hold on the tissues. Work on the far (contralateral) side of the abdomen, then swap sides.

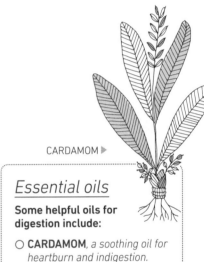

CARDAMOM ▶

Essential oils

Some helpful oils for digestion include:

○ **CARDAMOM**, *a soothing oil for heartburn and indigestion.*

○ **PEPPERMINT** *to calm indigestion and pep up sluggish digestion.*

○ **GINGER** *for its deeply soothing effect on digestion, especially with stress-related upset.*

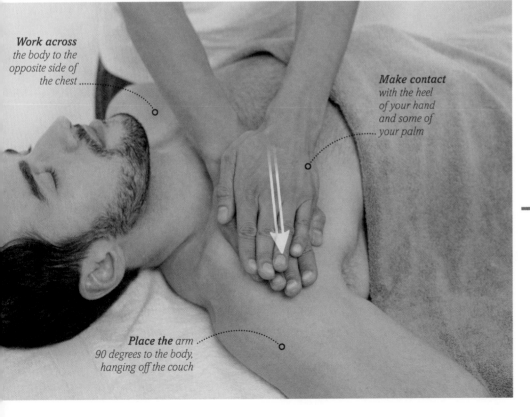

Work across the body to the opposite side of the chest

Make contact with the heel of your hand and some of your palm

Place the arm 90 degrees to the body, hanging off the couch

OPENING THE CHEST

◀ **Working at a computer** can create a C-shaped posture that compresses internal organs and compromises digestion. Try this opening technique. Place reinforced hands midchest and glide deeply out to the top of the arm to stretch out muscles and relieve tension. Work very slowly, watching the receiver's face for a reaction. Repeat on the opposite side.

MENSTRUAL COMPLAINTS

Working on the abdomen during menstruation can be very soothing, helping warm the tissues and ease cramping. The key is to use light pressure only during this time, avoiding vigorous movements and working softly and smoothly, using just effleurage movements when the abdomen is sensitive. Gentle effleurage on the legs, which can feel heavy and dragging, can also be beneficial.

BASIC TECHNIQUES USED:
○ **Circle strokes, p.46**
○ **Slide and glide, p.44**

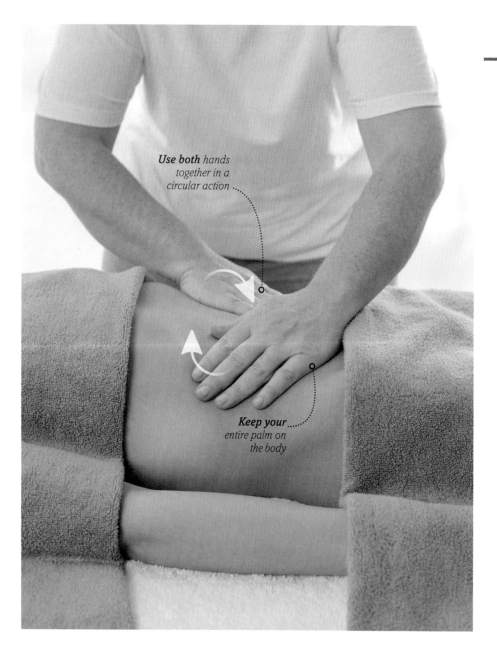

Use both hands together in a circular action

Keep your entire palm on the body

SOOTHING THE ABDOMEN

◀ **Gentle effleurage** over the abdomen warms and soothes the tissues to help ease menstrual cramps and discomfort. Circle lightly and extremely slowly over the area with both hands, making just small rotations and avoiding pushing up strongly into the ribs.

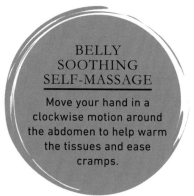

BELLY
SOOTHING
SELF-MASSAGE

Move your hand in a clockwise motion around the abdomen to help warm the tissues and ease cramps.

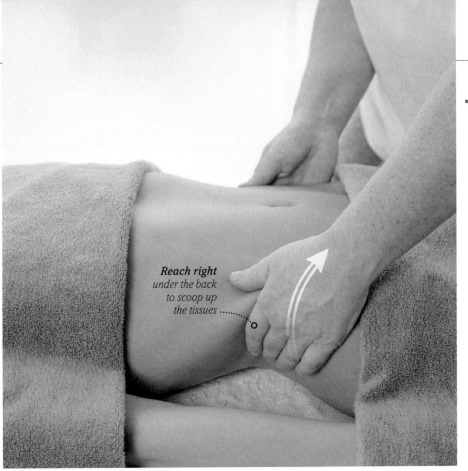

Reach right under the back to scoop up the tissues

LOWER BACK RELEASE

◀ **Lower back pain** can often accompany abdominal cramps, as contractions cause pain to radiate out from the abdomen. Pulling up tissues from the back while the receiver lies face up helps release and soothe the muscles around the back without putting pressure on the abdomen.

Essential oils

Some helpful oils for menstrual complaints include:

○ **GERANIUM** *to balance emotions and acts as a diuretic.*

○ **ROSE** *for its soothing effect.*

○ **CARDAMOM**, *an antispasmodic, helpful for digestive bloating.*

GERANIUM ▶

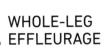

Keeping your outside hand in front lets you work up the whole leg

WHOLE-LEG EFFLEURAGE

◀ **Effleuraging** the whole leg can counter the dragging feeling that can be experienced here during menstruation. This stimulates blood flow, freshening the legs, and helps flush out waste to reduce fluid retention. Use the dragon's mouth slide and glide technique, shown here, or other effleurage strokes.

ANXIETY

Chronic anxiety creates tension throughout the body. In particular, it can cause palpitations, rapid breathing, and digestive complaints. A whole-body massage, with added focus on relaxing effleurage strokes and homing in on areas of concern, helps the receiver to let go and release emotional tension so you can work deeply into the tissues.

BASIC TECHNIQUES USED:
○ **Static pressures, p.72**
○ **Circle strokes, p.46**
○ **Deep strokes, p.52**
○ **Slide and glide, p.44**
○ **Thousand hands, p.42**
○ **Fan stroke, p.40**

▌GENTLE CHEST-OPENING HOLD

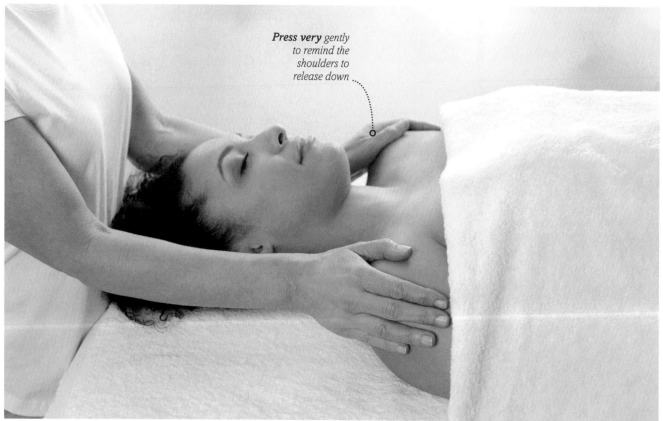

Press very gently to remind the shoulders to release down

▲ **Placing your hands** on the shoulders and gently pressing down helps open up the chest area, which can calm breathing and encourage the receiver to let go and relax. If the receiver feels anxious about placing their head in the face hold, this can be a gentle way to start a session and introduce your touch.

Essential oils

Some helpful oils for anxiety include:

○ **LAVENDER**, *which has a profoundly relaxing effect, helping ease anxiety.*

○ **NEROLI** *for its balancing and reviving properties.*

○ **FRANKINCENSE** *to lift the spirits, helping improve focus and balance energy.*

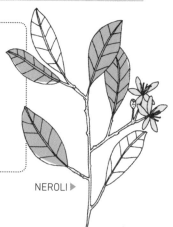

NEROLI ▶

ABDOMINAL EFFLEURAGE

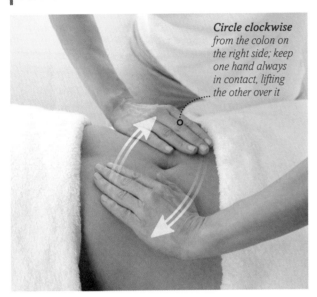

Circle clockwise from the colon on the right side; keep one hand always in contact, lifting the other over it

▲ **Anxiety often manifests** as digestive upset. Gentle effleurage helps stimulate abdominal tissues and aid peristalsis to boost digestion. Work fairly gently here and for quite a long time.

WORKING INTO THE DIAPHRAGM

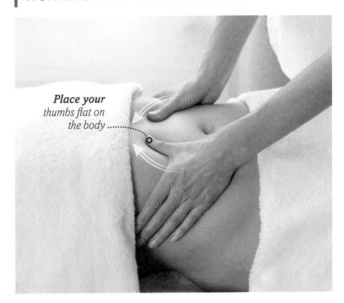

Place your thumbs flat on the body

▲ **Place your thumbs** below the ribs, then push up into the diaphragm to deepen breathing. Follow the receiver's breathing, applying deeper pressure on their out breath. Work sensitively, lightening pressure if you feel resistance.

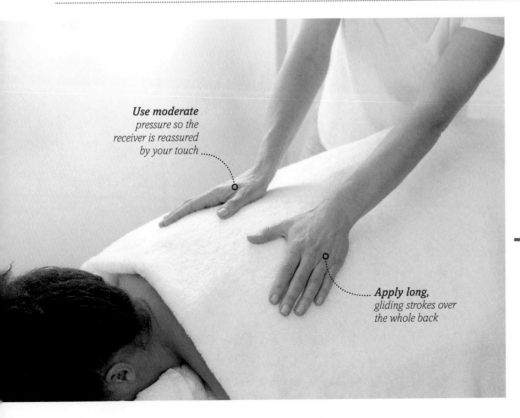

Use moderate pressure so the receiver is reassured by your touch

Apply long, gliding strokes over the whole back

CALMING SELF-MASSAGE

To focus your breathing, place your hands gently on your belly, relax, and observe your body pushing up into the hands with each breath.

CALMING BACK STROKES

◀ **Working over a towel** helps introduce touch gently to the back. Massage for a little while in this way with strokes you will return to later—such as thousand hands and fanning—to calm the receiver, put them in touch with their body, and allow them to feel safe before uncovering them.

DEPRESSION

The state of feeling low over a long period of time can manifest in many ways, including a loss of interest in events, tearfulness, feeling sluggish, and an inability to focus. The aim with massage is to stimulate circulation and revitalize body and mind, using vigorous techniques and energizing strokes—checking that the receiver is comfortable. Include fast, dynamic effleurage and lively petrissage, as well as the energizing, speedier percussion and reassuring stretching movements shown here.

BASIC TECHNIQUES USED:
○ **Percussion, p.64**
○ **Stretches, p.74**
○ **Shaking, p.68**
○ **Thousand hands, p.42**
○ **Rocking, p.70**

| PERCUSSION

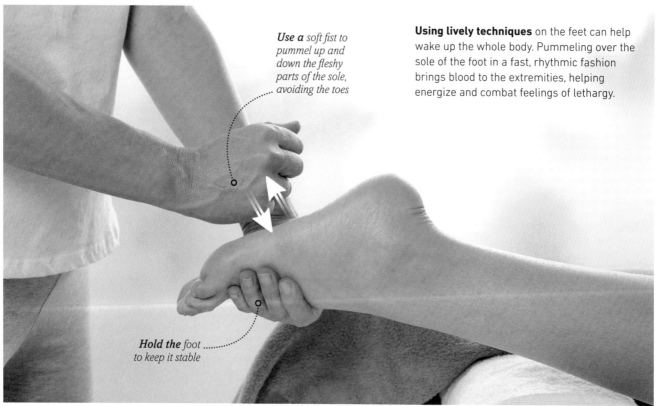

Use a soft fist to pummel up and down the fleshy parts of the sole, avoiding the toes

Using lively techniques on the feet can help wake up the whole body. Pummeling over the sole of the foot in a fast, rhythmic fashion brings blood to the extremities, helping energize and combat feelings of lethargy.

Hold the foot to keep it stable

Essential oils

Some helpful oils for depression include:

○ **ROSEMARY**, *a reviving oil that stimulates the nerves, improves focus, and helps combat feelings of lethargy.*

○ **MAY CHANG**, *which has calming, uplifting properties, helping quell feelings of panic.*

○ **BERGAMOT**—*its uplifting aroma acts as an antidepressant.*

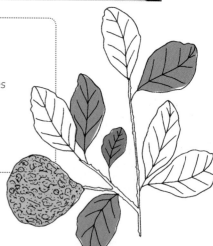

BERGAMOT ▶

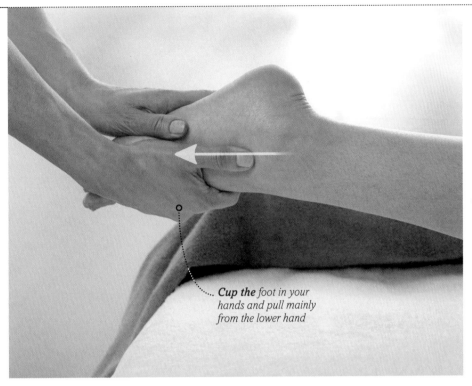

Cup the foot in your hands and pull mainly from the lower hand

STRETCHING LIMBS

◀ **Gently pulling** and extending a limb gives a sense that the body is being stretched and elongated, which helps the receiver to feel connected and present. You can gently shake the limb, too, before pulling to help energize the body. Leg pulls can be done with the receiver either prone or supine, and arm pulls done while supine.

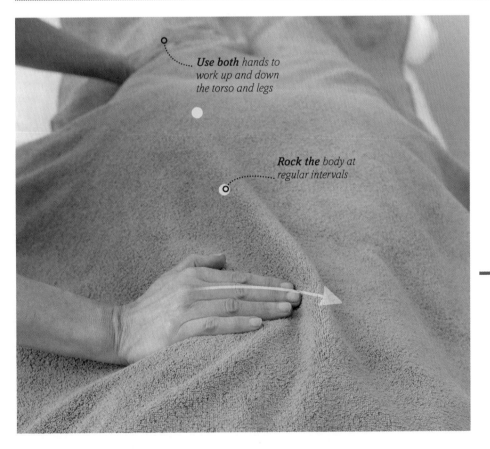

Use both hands to work up and down the torso and legs

Rock the body at regular intervals

REVITALIZING SELF-MASSAGE

Try some lively thousand hands effleurage on the thighs to wake up the tissues and boost circulation.

STIMULATING ROCKING

◀ **Once the session** is drawing to a close or you have finished working on one side and have covered the receiver with a towel, rocking the whole body fairly vigorously helps bring the receiver back into a greater state of awareness, awakening the body and mind.

LOW VITALITY

Low vitality can be due to factors such as convalescence, illness, or fatigue and may be accompanied by issues such as loss of appetite and insomnia. Your approach is important here; for example, if someone is frail, a 1-hour massage may be too long. Communication is also key, especially if making a home visit, and essential oil blends (see pp.24–29) may need to be weak in case of hypersensitivity.

BASIC TECHNIQUES USED:
○ **Slide and glide, p.44**

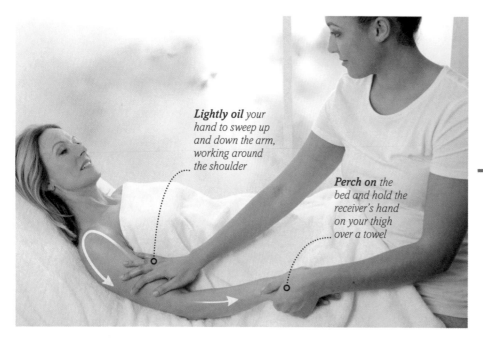

Lightly oil your hand to sweep up and down the arm, working around the shoulder

Perch on the bed and hold the receiver's hand on your thigh over a towel

GENTLE EFFLEURAGE

◄ **Using lots of soothing** effleurage relaxes the receiver deeply to help deal with issues such as insomnia. A gentler, less vigorous approach is ideal, maybe focusing on the upper body if doing a short massage, with the receiver propped up. Talk to them as you work, checking how the pressure feels.

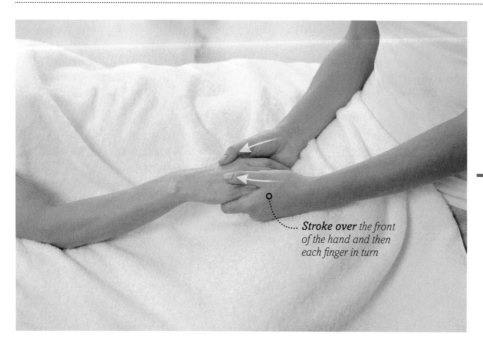

Stroke over the front of the hand and then each finger in turn

STROKING THE HAND

◄ **Very light stroking** of the hand while you perch on the bed can be extremely soothing and a good area to focus on if, for example, someone is unwell and doesn't wish to have a whole-body massage. Make sure the areas you aren't working on are well covered to keep the receiver warm.

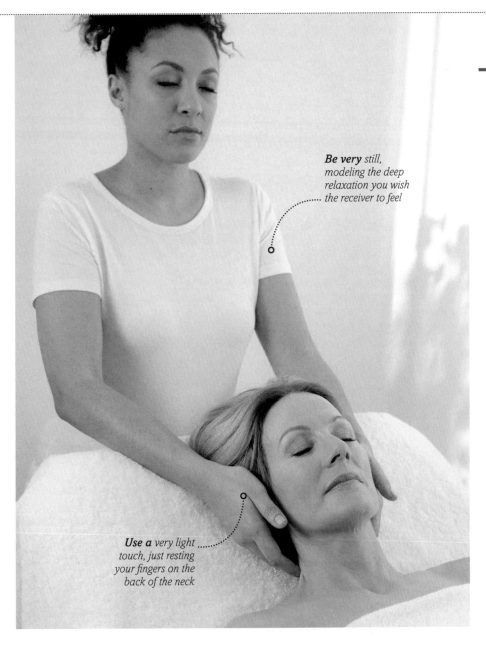

Be very still, modeling the deep relaxation you wish the receiver to feel

Use a very light touch, just resting your fingers on the back of the neck

RELAXING HEAD HOLD

◀ **Gently cupping** the back of the head is a very subtle technique that works on the autonomic nervous system (see p.20), orienting the receiver to a state of deep relaxation. Do this either at the start or to finish a session, when you can feel for signs of vitality and healing. As you hold the head, sense the movement of fluids and the softening of fascia. This can also be done on the feet.

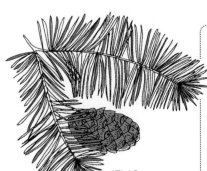

ATLAS ◀ CEDARWOOD

Essential oils

Some helpful oils for low vitality include:

○ **ATLAS CEDARWOOD**, *which has an uplifting effect, helping remove feelings of lethargy.*

○ **FRANKINCENSE** *for its soothing aroma that is calming, uplifting, and revitalizing.*

○ **PATCHOULI**, *which has antidepressant and grounding actions that help increase feelings of well-being.*

FIBROMYALGIA

This chronic condition causes widespread pain and can be accompanied by chronic fatigue and general stiffness. The causes are unknown, but it has been linked to prior viral infections and anxiety. Massage should be slow and gentle, being guided by the receiver on how much they can tolerate. Work is done on trigger points, all of which are affected; as the level of pain can be acute, these should be worked on with care.

BASIC AND OTHER TECHNIQUES USED:
- ○ **Static pressure, p.72**
- ○ **Trigger point therapy, p.130**

| RELEASING TENSION IN THE TRAPEZIUS

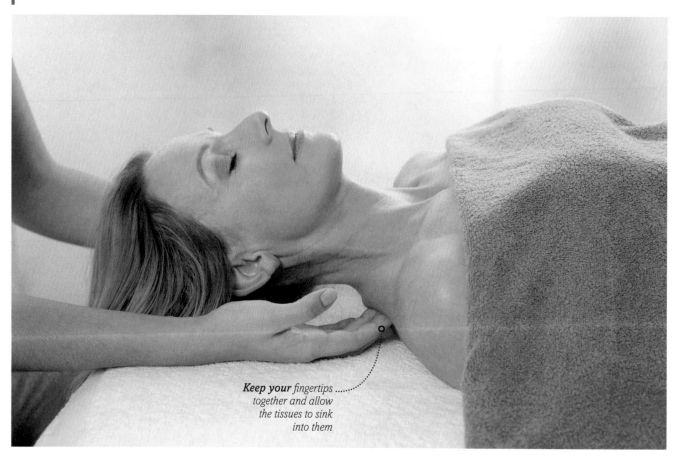

Keep your fingertips *together and allow the tissues to sink into them*

▲ **This static pressure** works into the trapezius muscles, which are generally very tense. As you place your hands under the top of the trapezius in the back, your fingers work into the trigger points, but this must be done with sensitivity. Gauge the receiver's response, and if the tissues allow and pain isn't too intense, push up into the tissues a bit more.

Essential oils

Some helpful oils for fibromyalgia include:

- ○ **LAVENDER** *for its mild painkilling properties.*
- ○ **FRANKINCENSE** *for its tonic and warming action.*
- ○ **ATLAS CEDARWOOD** *for its warming properties that help relieve pain and discomfort.*

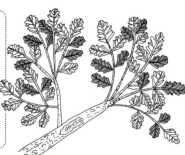

FRANKINCENSE ▶

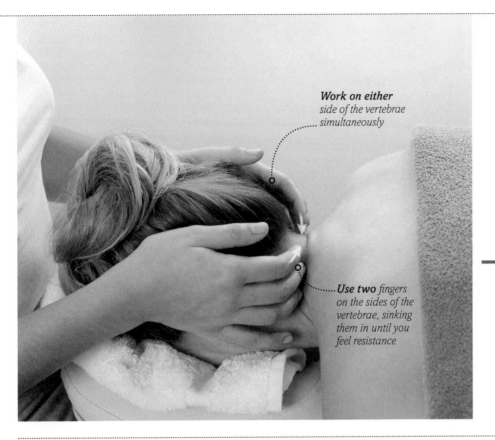

Work on either side of the vertebrae simultaneously

Use two fingers on the sides of the vertebrae, sinking them in until you feel resistance

RELEASING TENSION IN THE NECK

◀ **The area around** the cervical vertebrae in the neck can be inflamed and painful in everyone as fluids congest. With fibromyalgia, you need to work into this area even more gently. Sink your fingers in on one spot, then wait for release before pressing a bit more if the tissues allow.

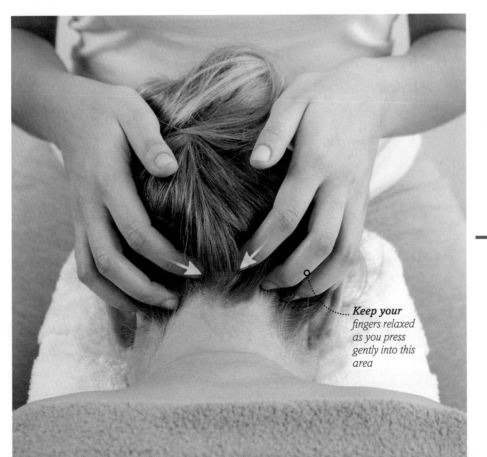

Keep your fingers relaxed as you press gently into this area

PRESSURE POINT WORK ON THE SKULL

◀ **The base of the skull**—the occipital ridge—has an important acupressure point on either side of the cervical vertebrae that is often painful, so it is important to work into. Working on this area while the receiver is face down allows you to control the pressure to ensure it is not too strong.

TAILORING TREATMENTS
MASSAGE FOR CLIENT GROUPS

Massage should always be tailored to meet the individual's needs on any given day. There are also certain stages or times of life when adaptations to massage practice are needed to meet the requirements of particular groups of people. Massage for babies requires just a light touch, with emphasis placed on the bonding opportunity, as well as on actual techniques. In pregnancy and old age, or in times of illness or where there is reduced mobility, thought needs to be given to your massage approach and adjustments made to ensure comfort. Knowing how to adapt your practice can help ensure you provide a truly holistic and therapeutic massage for each person.

PREGNANCY

A whole-body massage during pregnancy can be a wonderfully relaxing experience, with adapted positions and pillows for support ensuring comfort. Generally, pressure is a little lighter, but not so light as to be ticklish, and percussive techniques are avoided, keeping the focus on relaxation. Check if the receiver is happy for her abdomen to be touched; if she is, then this is perfectly safe. More treatment-oriented pregnancy massage to support medical treatments for particular pregnancy concerns and conditions requires specialty training.

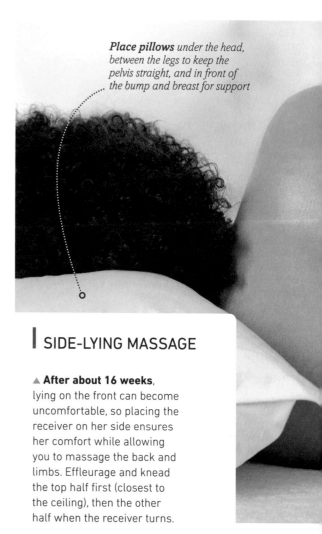

Place pillows under the head, between the legs to keep the pelvis straight, and in front of the bump and breast for support

SIDE-LYING MASSAGE

▲ **After about 16 weeks**, lying on the front can become uncomfortable, so placing the receiver on her side ensures her comfort while allowing you to massage the back and limbs. Effleurage and knead the top half first (closest to the ceiling), then the other half when the receiver turns.

BASIC TECHNIQUES USED:
- ○ **Slide and glide, p.44**
- ○ **Kneading, p.60**
- ○ **Criss-cross, p.48**
- ○ **Circle strokes, p.46**

WORKING ON THE HAND WHILE SIDE-LYING

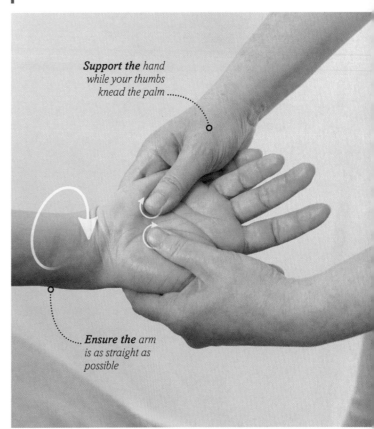

Support the hand *while your thumbs knead the palm* ⋯⋯

Ensure the arm *is as straight as possible*

▲ **To massage the hand** while the receiver lies on her side, you need to turn it backward, in a clockwise direction. This feels counterintuitive but is the only way to access the palm in this position.

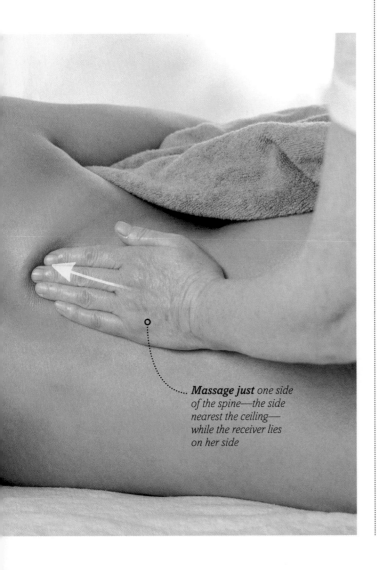

⋯ *Massage just* one side of the spine—the side nearest the ceiling— while the receiver lies on her side

Essential oils

The following are all safe for use in pregnancy:

- ○ **MANDARIN** *is a calming and uplifting oil.*
- ○ **PALMAROSA** *is a balancing and reviving oil.*
- ○ **LAVENDER** *is deeply relaxing, helping to promote rest and relaxation.*

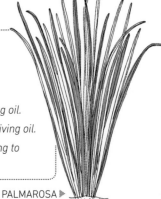

PALMAROSA ▶

CONTINUED ▶

PREGNANCY *continued*

| ELEVATED MASSAGE

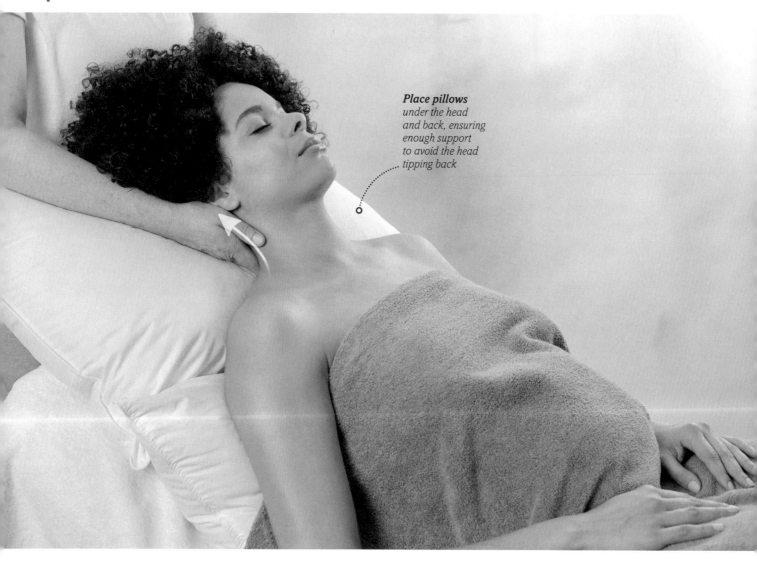

Place pillows
*under the head
and back, ensuring
enough support
to avoid the head
tipping back*

▲ **As the pregnancy bump** grows, lying on the back becomes uncomfortable and can cause dizziness as the baby presses on the vena cava. Raising the upper half of the body, keeping the head higher than the heart, keeps the receiver comfortable while you massage the upper body. Use pillows to build support, with a pillow under the thighs, too, to lift the pelvis.

"Pillows provide support and ensure comfort when raising the upper half of the body."

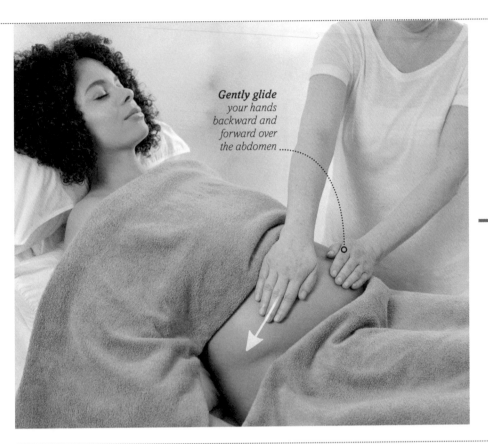

Gently glide your hands backward and forward over the abdomen

ABDOMINAL MASSAGE

◄ **Working on the abdomen**, if the receiver is happy for you to do so, is safe during all the trimesters and can be extremely relaxing. Your aim is for a gentle massage here, and the taut skin will mean you won't be working deeply. Try a criss-cross effleurage on the lower abdomen, as shown here, or circle in a clockwise motion, starting with small circles and then making them bigger.

ACCESSING THE LOWER LEG

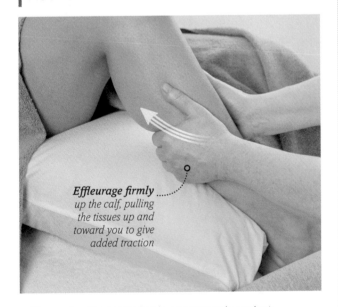

Effleurage firmly up the calf, pulling the tissues up and toward you to give added traction

▲ **Massaging the lower leg** in pregnancy is easiest with the receiver face up, leg bent, as it's hard to access this area when side-lying. Perch on the bed and sit on the foot, ideally over a towel, to anchor it.

SEATED MASSAGE

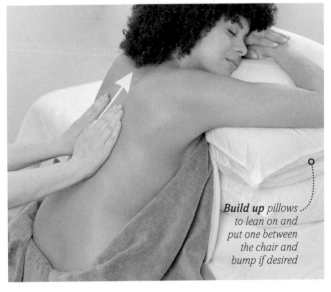

Build up pillows to lean on and put one between the chair and bump if desired

▲ **Sitting astride a chair**, leaning into a bed, gives access to the whole back and is helpful for partners who wish to offer supportive massage in pregnancy and labor. Feet should be flat on the floor to avoid the chair digging into the thigh.

BABY MASSAGE

Baby massage uses touch to communicate, applying soft, rhythmic strokes while you talk, sing, and make eye contact with your baby. Babies can be massaged at any age, although often parents begin at around 6 weeks. As your baby grows accustomed to massage, he will start to anticipate your touch, in turn enhancing your bond. Choose a time when your baby is quietly alert and start with short 10-minute sessions, building up time if he enjoys massage. Make sure the room is warm and that your baby has a comfortable, safe surface—a changing mat on the floor covered by a towel is ideal. Try the simple sequence here to introduce your baby to massage, lightly oiling your hands to apply gentle yet firm strokes and avoiding deep pressure or a too-light touch that could tickle.

WHEN NOT TO MASSAGE

There are certain times to avoid baby massage. These are just after a feeding; if your baby has a fever; for 24–48 hours after vaccines; and if your baby is tired, hungry, or irritable.

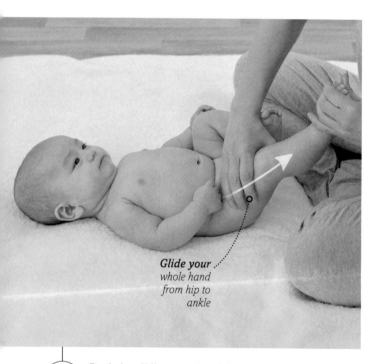

Glide your whole hand from hip to ankle

(1) **Begin by gliding your hand** down the leg to warm the tissues and introduce your touch. Starting on the legs is familiar and reassuring, as your baby is used to these being handled during diaper changes.

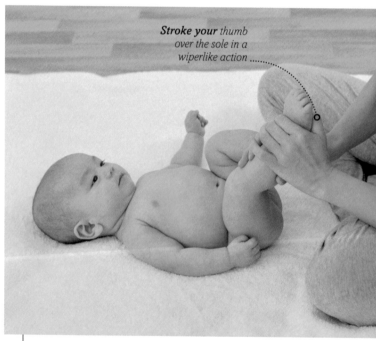

Stroke your thumb over the sole in a wiperlike action

(2) **Support the leg** and stroke your thumb over the foot, from heel to toe, alternating thumbs. The toes may splay out as you are stimulating the newborn plantar reflex here. Stroke back down the leg.

Useful oils

Some helpful oils for baby massage include:

○ **COLD-PRESSED VEGETABLE OILS** *such as sunflower or olive oil. Avoid nut-based oils and all essential oils.*

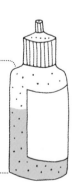

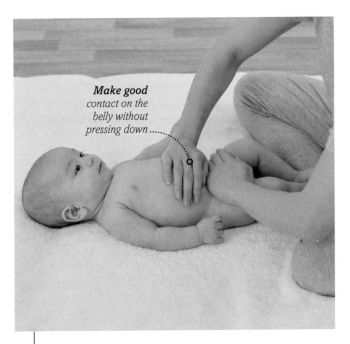

Make good contact on the belly without pressing down

3 **Put your hands** one above the other on the belly, palms flat, the higher hand just below the ribs. Now slide the hands toward the groin, one following the other.

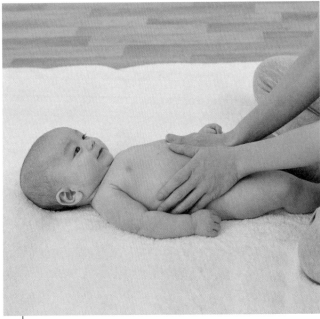

4 **Slide both hands** out to the sides, so that your thumbs point up to the head and your fingers hold the side of the body. Repeat steps 3 and 4 several times.

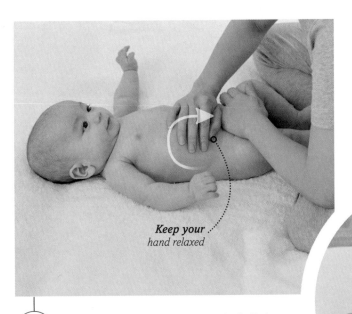

Keep your hand relaxed

5 **Glide your hand** clockwise over the belly in a semicircle. Place one hand gently over the groin to stop the legs kicking up. Position your other hand at the "7 o'clock" point on the abdomen, then sweep it around to the "5 o'clock" position, making a rainbow shape.

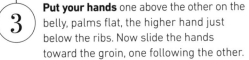

◀ **COLIC SOOTHER**
Alternating the rainbow sweep with gentle leg bounces relaxes the belly to help ease colic. Repeat this several times.

CONTINUED ▶

BABY MASSAGE *continued*

"Hold your baby's gaze throughout the massage to enhance the loving bond between you."

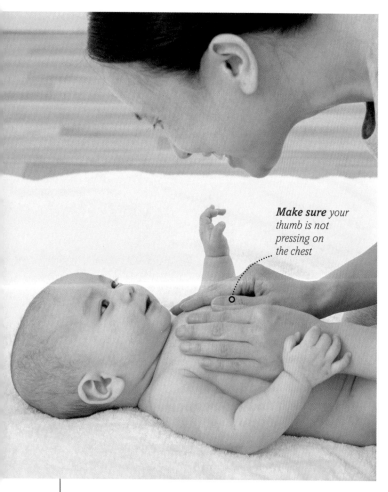

Make sure your thumb is not pressing on the chest

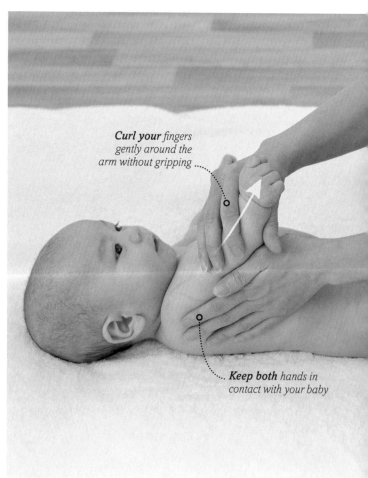

Curl your fingers gently around the arm without gripping

Keep both hands in contact with your baby

(6) **Move to the upper chest.** Gently place your hands on the chest area, then sweep them out over the chest. Come in close as you make this action and smile and talk to your baby, keeping eye contact all the while.

(7) **Gently hold the arm** and sweep down with your fingers, from the shoulder all the way to the fingertips. Take care not to pull the limb as you make this move. This downward action is a relaxing one for your baby.

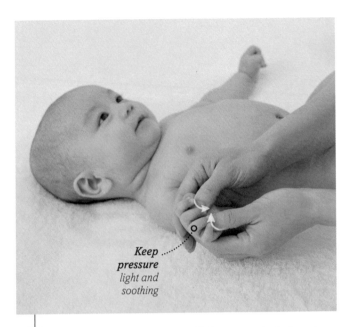

Keep pressure light and soothing

8 **Gently massage the hand.** Using one or both thumbs, circle over the palm, working inward and outward as feels natural. The fingers will naturally curl in. Finish with a stimulating sweep up the arm, then repeat steps 7 and 8 on the opposite arm.

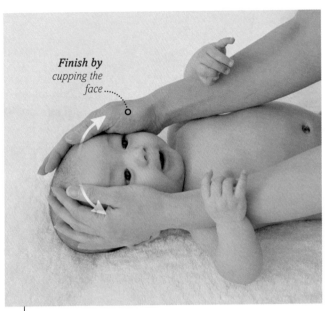

Finish by cupping the face

9 **Move to the face.** Rest both hands on the top of the forehead, then stroke your thumbs out over the forehead, gently resting your fingers on the head as you do so and avoiding covering the eyes with your hands.

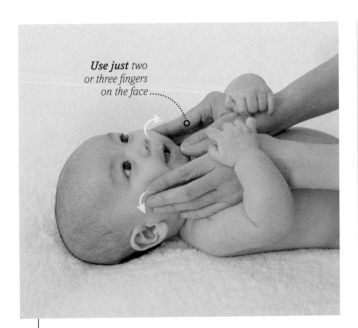

Use just two or three fingers on the face

10 **Circle gently over the cheeks** using the pads of your fingers, circling outward with both hands. Start near the mouth and work out toward the ears. Keep your fingers relaxed all the time to avoid transferring any tension to your baby.

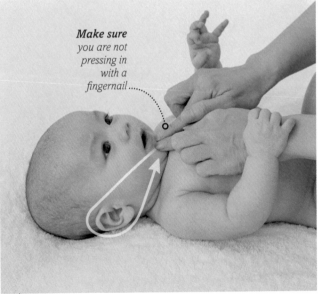

Make sure you are not pressing in with a fingernail

11 **Position your index fingers** in the center of the chin. Stroke each finger out across the face, traveling up to the ear, then circling the ear and stroking back to the chin. This is particularly soothing for teething and earaches.

CONTINUED ▶

BABY MASSAGE *continued*

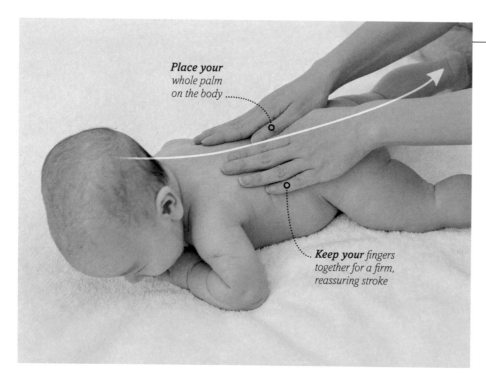

Place your whole palm on the body

Keep your fingers together for a firm, reassuring stroke

If your baby is happy on his front, turn him over for a quick massage on the back of his body. Younger babies may only be happy to spend a few minutes on their front, so be guided by your baby. Sweep your hands all the way down the body, from the back of the head, down the back and legs, and over the feet, in one big gliding stroke.

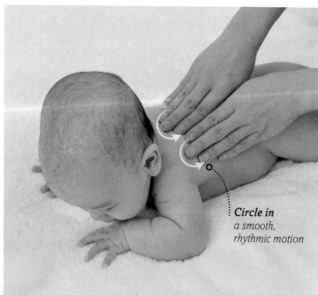

Circle in a smooth, rhythmic motion

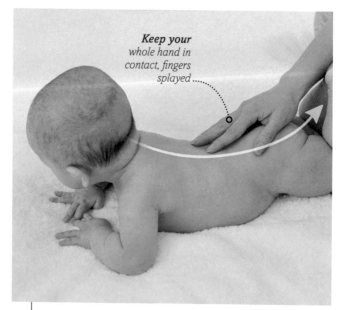

Keep your whole hand in contact, fingers splayed

13 **Use your fingertips** to make light circles down the back, working on either side of the spine. Make small, counterclockwise circles with the fingers, working down one side of the back, avoiding the spine, then moving over to the other side of the spine to repeat.

14 **Close your massage** with soothing "combing" strokes down the whole of the body, keeping your fingers separated and alternating your hands as you stroke down from head to feet several times.

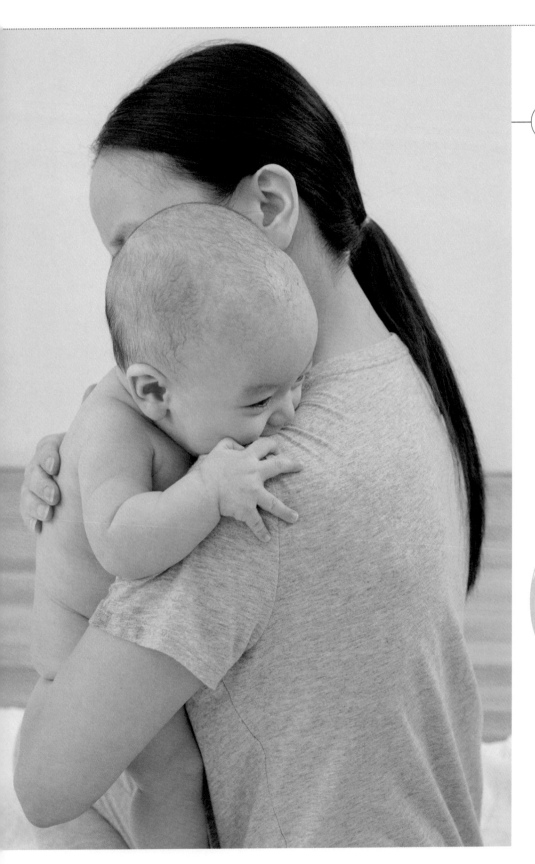

15

Once you've finished, pick up your baby right away and enjoy a cuddle, savoring the bonding experience you've shared. Place a towel around him if you wish for a moment, then dress him to keep him warm and relaxed.

DEEPENING THE BOND

Parents who regularly massage their baby report greater confidence in handling them and say that massage helps them to feel more in tune with their baby's needs.

MASSAGE FOR OLDER PEOPLE

The holistic benefits of massage apply to all, but for older people, the benefits can be profound, improving circulation and muscle tone where there is inactivity and providing nurturing touch where this is lacking. Adaptations may be made: if the receiver prefers to be clothed, a chair massage is ideal, and a massage may be brief if a person is frail. Generally, touch may be lighter, using oil to avoid friction on fragile skin.

BASIC AND OTHER TECHNIQUES USED:
○ **Kneading, p.60**
○ **Slide and glide, p.44**
○ **Indian head massage, p.164**

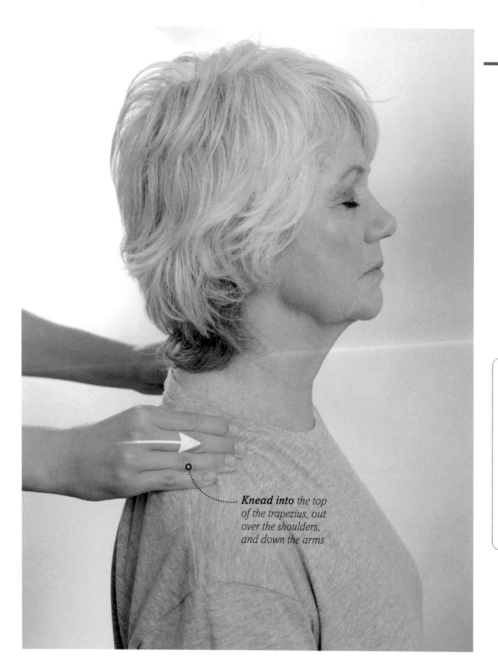

Knead into the top of the trapezius, out over the shoulders, and down the arms

UPRIGHT CHAIR MASSAGE

◀ **A chair massage** that allows you to work on the upper body can be ideal if the receiver would like to gain the benefits of touch without undressing for a whole-body massage. Try to ensure that your wrists are straight and relaxed and observe the receiver's response, adjusting pressure if needed.

Essential oils

Some helpful oils for older people include:

○ **ROSE** *for its calming and uplifting properties that help relax and soothe anxiety.*

○ **FRANKINCENSE,** *which increases energy and focus.*

○ **LAVENDER** *to condition and rejuvenate skin.*

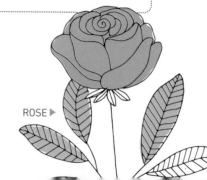

ROSE ▶

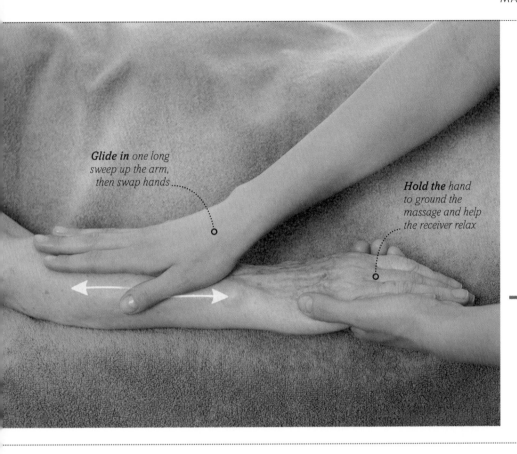

Glide in one long sweep up the arm, then swap hands

Hold the hand to ground the massage and help the receiver relax

SOOTHING ARM EFFLEURAGE

◀ **If you are giving** a shorter massage, you may wish to focus mainly on the upper body. Long, gliding arm effleurage can be very soothing and warming, helping revitalize and tone muscles.

RELAXING HAND MASSAGE

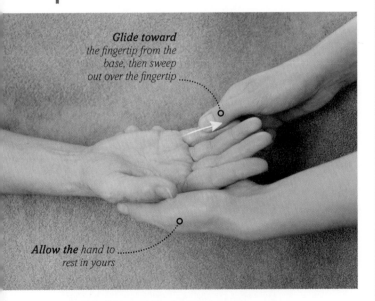

Glide toward the fingertip from the base, then sweep out over the fingertip

Allow the hand to rest in yours

▲ **The hand is easily accessible,** and massage here very relaxing. If the skin is thin and the veins prominent on the front of the hand, focus on the palm, kneading it, then stroking each finger in turn.

FACIAL STROKES

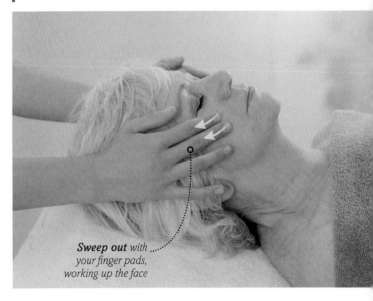

Sweep out with your finger pads, working up the face

▲ **Gently stroking the face** can be intensely soothing, and you can raise the bed a little if this feels more comfortable for the receiver. Keep pressure light, again being mindful of fragile skin.

REDUCED MOBILITY

Mobility may be limited for a number of reasons, including disability and a prolonged period of recovery after surgery. When mobility is reduced, the circulation can become sluggish and muscle tone may be gradually lost as muscles are underused. Massage is a helpful tool to stimulate the tissues, helping improve circulation and revitalize muscles, though it should be avoided in the period immediately after surgery.

BASIC TECHNIQUES USED:
○ **Rotations, p.76**
○ **Slide and glide, p.44**

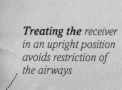

Treating the receiver in an upright position avoids restriction of the airways

Support the hand so it can completely let go

Guide the arm in small circles from the elbow, making small rotations

MOBILIZING JOINTS

▲ **If someone is sedentary** for a great deal of time—for example, when using a wheelchair—the arms can stiffen. Moving them in small, passive rotations helps release tension in the joints and improve muscle tone. Effleurage the arm first to warm tissues, then rotate the arm in both directions both to facilitate movement and to increase the range of motion.

Essential oils

Some helpful oils for reduced mobility include:

○ **MAY CHANG**, *which improves circulation and has an uplifting effect.*

○ **BLACK PEPPER** *and* **ROSEMARY** *to stimulate circulation and clear congested airways.*

ROSEMARY ▶

STIMULATING TISSUES

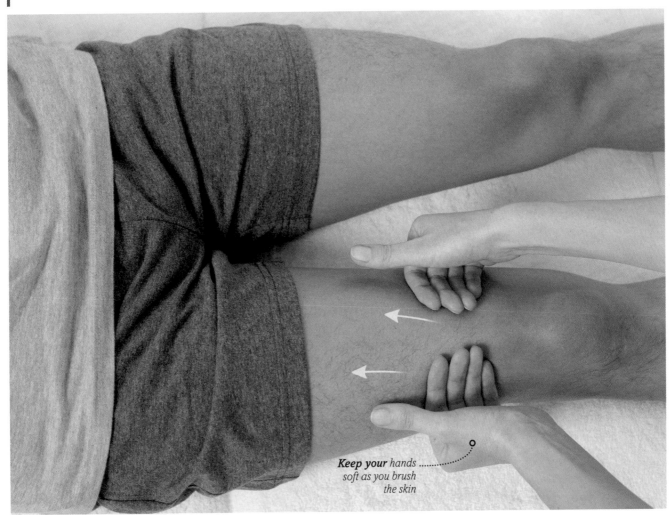

Keep your hands soft as you brush the skin

▲ **To improve circulation** and encourage the drainage of fluids in the legs, you can use the backs of your hands in a "skin-brushing" action along the thigh. No oil is needed for this. Keep pressure light and make small, brushing movements with your fingers up the thigh, using either both hands together or alternating hands.

CANCER SUPPORT

As with any illness, when massaging someone with cancer, think about their needs on that day. Avoid massaging over an area that has had recent surgery and avoid working over the affected area for 6 weeks after radiotherapy. A shorter massage may be preferable, focusing on the limbs and head if a full-body massage is too much, while gentle touch can help overcome negative feelings about a part of the body. Essential oil blends should be weaker (1 percent dilution, see p.27) and avoided with nausea.

BASIC TECHNIQUES USED:
- Slide and glide, p.44
- Circle strokes, p.46

Essential oils

Some helpful oils to support a person with cancer include:

- **LEMON, FRANKINCENSE**, and **ROSE**, *uplifting oils, which can help support the immune system. Lemon is also antimicrobial.*

◄ LEMON

A COMFORTABLE POSITION

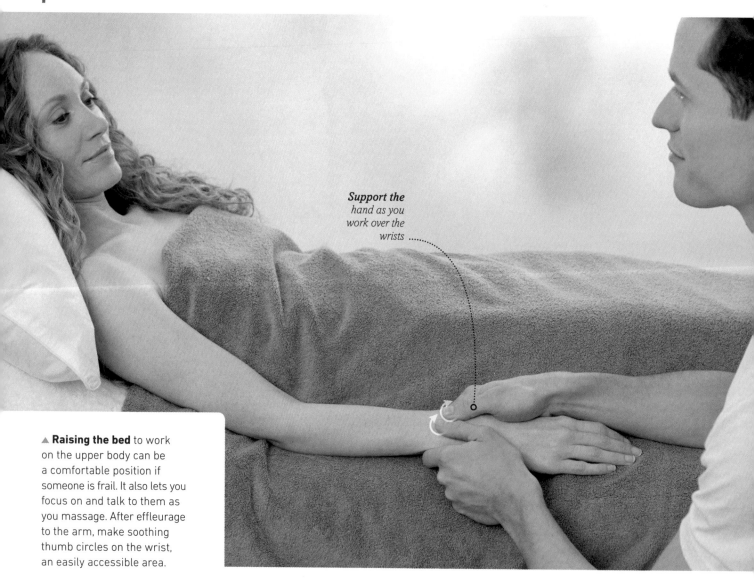

Support the hand as you work over the wrists ....

▲ **Raising the bed** to work on the upper body can be a comfortable position if someone is frail. It also lets you focus on and talk to them as you massage. After effleurage to the arm, make soothing thumb circles on the wrist, an easily accessible area.

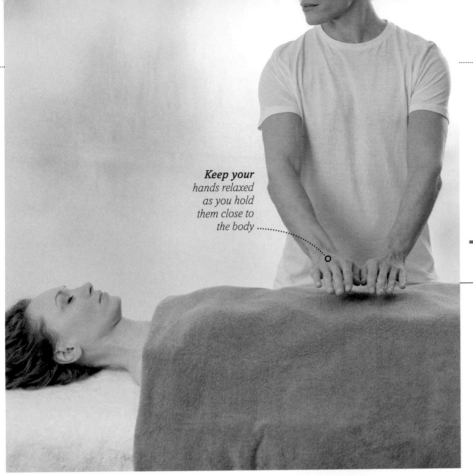

Keep your hands relaxed as you hold them close to the body ....

NURTURING TOUCH

If the receiver disassociates from an area after surgery, gentle contact over a towel can help them reconnect and feel comfortable with this part of the body again. Approach this with care. First, hover your hands over the area to sense energy before making any contact.

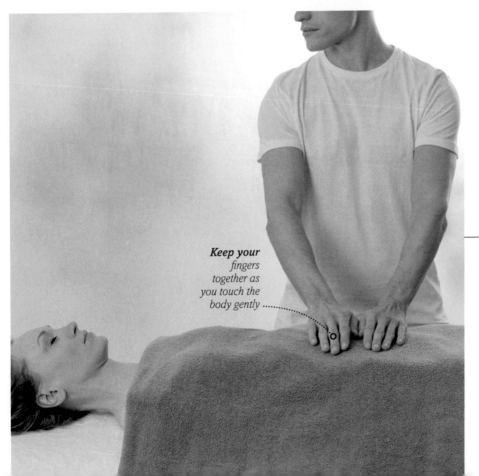

Keep your fingers together as you touch the body gently ....

2

Very slowly, lower your hands onto the body. No pressure is exerted here—it's just a gentle, warming touch. Stand straight so that you are not putting any body weight into the action, and rest your thighs against the couch. Watch the receiver and observe how her breathing relaxes.

GLOSSARY

Acupressure Effective form of stimulation by deep, firm pressure along acupuncture points to help relax muscles and free energy.

Aromatherapy Using aromatic plant extracts and essential oils for therapeutic purposes.

Autonomic nervous system The part of the body that involuntarily regulates internal functions. Made up of the sympathetic nervous system, parasympathetic nervous system, and enteric nervous system.

Ayurveda Traditional Indian holistic healing system based on the belief that health and wellness depend on balance between mind, body, and spirit.

Biodynamic massage Psychotherapeutic form of massage concerned with the integration of all aspects of an individual—physical, emotional, intellectual, and spiritual.

Cartilage The firm, flexible connective tissue found in human joints and other places such as the nose, throat, and ears.

Chakras Centers of spiritual power or energy that help regulate all the processes in the human body. Anatomically, they link to endocrine glands or nerve plexi (junctions).

Contralateral Relating to or denoting the other side of the body.

Deep tissue massage A type of massage therapy that focuses on realigning layers of muscle and connective tissue using slow, firm strokes and pressure.

Effleurage French for "touch lightly" or "skim," the gentle sliding stroke that relaxes the body and soft tissues.

Essential oil A concentrated, volatile oil extracted by distillation or expression from a botanical source.

Fascia Connective tissue that attaches, encloses, stabilizes, and separates muscles, nerves, blood vessels, and other internal organs.

Friction strokes Deep circular motions on the muscles to break down scar tissue and increase blood flow.

Holistic Treating a whole person rather than just a single symptom.

Hot stone therapy An ancient practice that involves the use of flat, heated stones to massage the body and promote deep relaxation.

Hypermobile Joints that can move beyond the normal range of motion.

Insertion point The point of attachment in a muscle where more movement occurs.

Involuntary muscle A muscle that contracts without conscious control.

Ipsilateral Belonging to or occurring on the same side of the body.

Ligaments Bundles of tough, flexible connective tissue that connect one bone to an adjacent bone.

Lymphatic system A network of vessels in the body through which lymph drains from the tissues into the blood.

Manual lymphatic drainage A type of massage that stimulates the lymphatic system to encourage the flow of lymph.

Meridians According to Traditional Chinese Medicine (TCM), meridians are the pathways of energy that flow through the body.

Mucolytic A substance that dissolves thick mucus.

Muscle contraction When a muscle contracts and changes length, either shortening or lengthening, or produces tension but stays the same length.

Muscle energy technique (MET) Manual therapy that uses the muscle's own energy in the form of gentle contractions to relax and lengthen the muscle.

Palpation Using the sense of touch to examine the tissues of the body physically.

Parasympathetic nervous system The part of the nervous system that unconsciously regulates the body during rest and recuperation.

Percussion A massage technique involving rapid and repeated striking of the body.

Petrissage Strokes that squeeze, roll, and knead the muscles.

Phototoxicity Some essential oils contain compounds that increase the skin's reactivity to the sun's rays, meaning sunburn is more likely.

Pulsing *See* rocking.

Reflexology System of massage based on the theory that there are reflex points on the feet, hands, and head linked to every part of the body.

Rocking Rhythmic, rocking form of body work where the body is rocked in a soft, regular rhythm. Pulsing uses this technique.

Sen channels In Thai massage practice, the channels that energy flows through around the body.

Shiatsu Means "finger pressure" in Japanese. Also involves therapeutic bodywork based on the same principles as acupuncture, using kneading, pressing, soothing, tapping, and stretching techniques.

Skeletal muscle A muscle that is connected to the skeleton, which forms part of the mechanical system that moves the limbs and other parts of the body.

Static pressure Applying pressure at a particular point without any movement from the therapist.

Swedish massage Developed in Sweden, Swedish massage is known as a "classic" massage and employs remedial manipulative techniques such as effleurage, petrissage, vibration, friction, and tapotement.

Sympathetic nervous system Part of the autonomic nervous system that controls involuntary responses and is responsible for the body's "fight or flight" reaction.

Tapotement *See* percussion.

Tendons Flexible cord of strong collagen tissue attaching a muscle to a bone.

Tissues Part of a living thing that is made up of similar cells, meant to perform a specific function.

Trigger point therapy Involves the application of pressure to tender muscle tissue to relieve pain and dysfunction in other parts of the body.

Trigger points A hyperirritable spot found in skeletal muscle fascia.

Vibration massage A fine, gentle trembling movement performed with hands or fingers. Shaking massage movements also vibrate underlying tissues. Used to stimulate soft tissues in the body.

Voluntary muscle Muscle that is under conscious control and is generally attached to the skeleton.

RESOURCES

AROMATHERAPY

Aromatherapy Trade Council (ATC)
a-t-c.org
Information on essential oils.

Canadian Federation of Aromatherapists
cfacanada.com
Information on essential oils and training, as well as practitioners.

National Association for Holistic Aromatherapy
naha.org
Information on aromatherapy and essential oils.

Neal's Yard Remedies
us.nyorganic.com
Supplier of essential oils.
Email: inquiries.us@nyorganic.com
Tel: 888-NYR-0909

MASSAGE INFORMATION AND COURSES

American Massage Therapy Association
amtamassage.org
Details on courses and practitioners.

Massage Therapy in Canada
massage.ca
Information on practitioners, as well as schools and certification.

Acupuncture Canada
acupuncturecanada.org
Information on training, certification, and practitioners.

Chinese Medicine and Acupuncture Association of Canada
cmaac.ca
Find a practitioner; details on training.

American Reflexology Certification Board
arcb.net
Become certified as a reflexologist.

American Society of Acupuncturists
asacu.org
Find a practitioner of acupuncture and East Asian medicine.

Associated Bodywork and Massage Professionals
abmp.com
Find practitioners; learn about certification.

Ayurvedic Institute
ayurveda.com
Ayurvedic practitioner training; spa.

Ayurveda Association of Canada
ayurvedaassociation.ca
Find a practitioner; details on events.

National Association of Myofascial Trigger Point Therapists
myofascialtherapy.org
Association for professionals who practice trigger-point therapy.

Reflexology Association of America
reflexology-usa.org
Information on reflexology and courses.

Reflexology Association of Canada
reflexologycanada.org
Find a practitioner; information on training and certification.

Vodder School of Manual Lymphatic Drainage
vodderschool.com
Organization representing manual lymphatic drainage (MLD) practitioners from the Dr. Vodder school of MLD. Information on courses.

INDEX

ACKNOWLEDGMENTS

VICTORIA PLUM WOULD LIKE TO GIVE THE FOLLOWING THANKS:

First, I would like to thank Robert Tisserand, in many ways the father and early ambassador of English aromatherapy. It was Robert's reach that introduced me to the essential oils at the start, and through the oils that I discovered the power of touch, in their application. A continuing inspiration is my friend and colleague who teaches massage, Elaine Tomkins. Many conversations, deep and informative, about this therapy continue my growth. Most of all, thanks are due to my clients over the years, who helpfully demonstrate what I don't know and make me study to be better. And to my students, asking me questions that I can't answer and inspiring me through this.

Working on this book has been a wonderful challenge: Claire Cross, as editor, questioning me about what I am doing and why I am doing it as we worked together in the studio or looked at pictures and text, made me go back to asking myself those useful questions again and reinforced my passion and purpose in the work. Louise Brigenshaw rose to the challenge of translating dynamic movement through still photographs. Finally, Nigel Wright and Julie Stewart were a duo of delight, working with serious integrity—but bringing such fun into the space.

DK WOULD LIKE TO THANK:

The authors for their guidance and expertise throughout, and the following practitioners for their invaluable support and guidance: Emma Bond, Lisa Gwilliam, Simon Heale, Dee Jones, Jo Kellett, Esther Mason, Susan Mumford, Louise Robinson, Noriko Sakura, and Yunfeng Wu.

Photography assistant Julie Stewart
Photography coordinator Janice Browne
Makeup artist Victoria Barnes

Illustration Ryn Frank
Illustration and design Vanessa Hamilton
Proofreading Claire Wedderburn-Maxwell
Indexing Hilary Bird

A big thank you to our models:
Courtesy of Source Models: Lauren Clements-Hill, Hayley Thomas, Mei-Li Burnside, Louise Barton, Martin Mednidrov, Colin Lee, Stephanie Warren, Suzi Langhorne, Charles Ruhrmund

Courtesy of Elliott Brown Agency: Fiona Pemberton, Natalie Gayle, Janine Craig

Courtesy of IMM Agency: Ava Jones, Daniel Carr

Courtesy of Beautiful Bumps:
Tessa and Lewis Poon

Disclaimer